Also by Siegfied J. Kra, M.D.

CORONARY BYPASS SURGERY: WHO NEEDS IT?
AGING MYTHS: REVERSIBLE CAUSES OF MIND AND MEMORY LOSS
EXAMINE YOUR DOCTOR
IS SURGERY NECESSARY?

The Three-Legged Stallion

The Three-Legged Stallion

and Other Tales from a Doctor's Notebook

SIEGFRIED J. KRA, M.D.

W · W · Norton & Company · New York · London

Published simultaneously in Canada by Penguin Books Canada Ltd.,
2801 John Street, Markham, Ontario L3R1B4.
Printed in the United States of America.

The text of this book is composed in Aranta with
display type set in Fenice light. Composition and
manufacturing by The Haddon Craftsmen, Inc.
Book design by Antonina Krass.

First Edition

Library of Congress Cataloging-in-Publication Data

Kra, Siegfried J.
    The Three-Legged Stallion and other Tales from a doctor's notebook / by
Siegfried J. Kra.
    p. cm.
    Contents: The three-legged stallion—Dead mackerel—The kosher connection—
The blue boater—The mad hatter—The man with the dark
sunglasses—Fever of unknown origin—Leysin—Night train to
Paris—The Marquise of Toulouse—The polo player—The yellow
light.
    1. Medicine—Miscellanea. I. Title.
R706.K72 1989
610—dc19

ISBN 0-393-02668-X   88-22572

W.W. Norton & Company, Inc.
500 Fifth Avenue, New York, N.Y. 10110
W.W. Norton & Company Ltd,
37 Great Russell Street, London WC1B 3NU
1 2 3 4 5 6 7 8 9 0

To Brigitte

All of the names as well as many of the identifying characteristics, details of background information, and incidents in these stories have been changed.

Contents

The
Three-Legged
Stallion

ONE

The Three-Legged Stallion

AMONGST HIS CRONIES he was called "the Stallion," but his mother had named him "Little Tony." How Little Tony became the Stallion is the essence of this tale.

Little Tony was born with little gray matter, but he had other qualities. He was very affable, athletic, and he had a very long penis. He was strikingly handsome with his long black hair and dashing black eyes, and he had a strong lean body that woman flocked to like bees to honey. His sexual capabilities became legendary even at an early age. Women of all ages yearned so for him that even in nearby villages his reputation spread. The boys of the town nicknamed him the Stallion. One drunken night they drove to a nearby city where a Spanish woman specialized in tattoos. She engraved a large red and brown three-legged stallion on Little Tony's chest, and when he walked on the beach in the summer, everyone knew who he was, especially the women. They would whisper and moan, "There goes the Stallion," as if he were a god who had come to this village for one main purpose.

The Stallion continued in this way, making very many women happy and grateful with his talent and natural endowment, until he reached the age of 45 when something terrible happened.

It was one of those marvelous nights under the stars when the Stallion was with a beautiful young blonde. After he finished all his endearing touches and sweet words, and was about to bring the young lady to her final ecstasy, his penis refused to respond. He tried everything and the girl tried everything, but it was no use. He was grateful she did not live in his town because how could he face up to the jeers and humiliation?

His nimble brain lined up the reasons for his failure: 1) the girl was too big; 2) the bed was too small; 3) the linguine was poisoned; 4) someone must have the evil eye on him. For the rest of the week, he searched faces for the evil eye, but found none.

He had heard the older men say, "Too much wine snuffs out the rod." For the next two weeks, he drank no alcohol, went to bed early, refrained from pumping iron, stopped smoking, and avoided coffee. Each night, he dreamt of being thrown into a deep pit with beautiful, naked women. He dreamt his erection was magnificent and tall and lasting, and more women had to be thrown into the well to fulfill his lust.

At the end of three weeks, well rested, decaffeinated, free of alcohol, he visited the most luscious gem of the town. The setting was marvelous—a sleazy motel with a large sagging bed surrounded by mirrors and red curtains. A torrid triple-X flick on the tube was the appetizer.

Margot was her name, she was a manicurist by trade, and she was so magnificent that she could raise the dead with her endless charms. The Stallion and the olive-skinned manicurist made a beautiful picture in bed. His excitement had never been greater, but his penis would have no part of it.

First came anger, then came depression and fear of future failures. Had he lost his one great asset in life? It might mean he would have to remove the Stallion and pin a pony on his chest.

Sleepless nights followed. He kept to himself and began to look haggard. He walked bent like the letter C, and his cronies began to wonder if he was not seriously ill. Maybe he was a fag. This thought made him shudder. He heard of macho guys who didn't know they were fags until they were 45 years old.

At his once-a-week poker game, Mano, the meat cutter, who looked like a bull, said, "You know Stallion, you don't look so good."

"I don't feel so good,"

Was it showing on his face, like hair growing on the palms of the hand if you did your own too much? He looked into the mirror and saw that his eyes looked old, the lids sagged, and his face had the color of cold spaghetti.

"I felt bad like you once. I took four Vitamin E pills every day, zinc, ginseng, and ground-up bull balls."

"Bull balls?"

"Yeah. When I was in Korea in the service, I had a girl who used to serve them to me if I was tired. You can't get them here, but the rest you can." He whispered, "I can make it four times a night if I want."

He left the poker game in great flight, exhilarated, and ran down to the local food store located next to the barber shop. He gulped down four Vitamin E's, four zinc pills, and ginseng. Although he got sick to his stomach, he did this for three days, and on the third night, he went to see Margot again but remained soft as putty.

There was no one to talk to him in his crisis until he picked up the New York newspaper that advertised help for men.

The word impotent made him feel sick to his stomach. The

advertisement read, "Sex therapist with surrogate for impotence and other problems." He didn't know what the word surrogate meant, but he made the appointment anyway.

The sex therapist was once a married housewife who had become a social worker specializing in sex problems. She listened to the sad tale and inquired all about his life as a child, his relationship with his mother and father, and even his great-aunt. She concluded that Little Tony had developed guilt feelings regarding women. Making love to women in many ways represented making love to his own mother.

To get rid of this mother's complex, Little Tony (he was no longer called the Stallion) was advised to see the social worker four times a week at $75 an hour. Little Tony had plenty of money because the numbers racket kept him quite affluent.

The surrogate turned out to be an insipid-looking woman who turned him inside out at each session, but nothing helped. All the cajoling and reassurance did not raise up his penis.

"You are not my mother, you are not my mother, you are not my mother," he repeated 1,000 times with each session.

At the end of three months, there was still no erection, and he decided to get a second opinion from a medical doctor. He told the doctor everything in his brain: "I smoke three packs of cigarettes per day, drink plenty, sniff cocaine twice a week, and feel physically excellent, except I can't get a hard-on. It's a disaster, Doctor. Do you see this?" and he pointed to the stallion on his chest. "I earned that name. You've got to help me. Money's no object."

"I can help you," the kindly doctor said. "What you need is B12 injections and hormones for three weeks, three times a week, at $25 an injection, and then your sex will return. Trust me."

He did.

After three more weeks, Little Tony's arm looked like it had suffered from smallpox, but he failed again with all the town prizes. His beard grew thicker and all his muscles bulged more than ever, except the one that meant the most to him. Desperate and crestfallen, he heard of a doctor in the next town, a diagnostician, a medical sleuth.

He parked his car and walked several blocks to the medical office. This was his last chance, he thought, and he became anxious. There is no life for a pony. His heart began to beat hard against his silk blue shirt. His hands trembled and became moist, and he noticed that his ankles began to ache as he climbed the hill toward the medical office.

The doctor asked him hundreds of questions, but all had "no" for an answer.

"The only thing that I noticed," he said, "is that I get pain in my calves after I walk a few blocks. Before, I could walk for hours doing my collections, now I can't even manage one-half block. I have to stop, wait until the pain leaves, and then I start to walk again. And my feet are always cold."

The doctor then asked the most important question. "Tony, do you wake up in the morning with a hard-on?"

"No," Tony answered, "not for the past three months."

This was the clue the doctor needed to determine the cause of this terrible problem that afflicted Tony. The doctor examined him from head to toe. He kept returning to feel the pulses in his groin. They were absent. The pulses on the top of his feet, called the pedal pulses, were absent. The pulses on the inside of his feet, called the tibial pulses, were gone. The doctor smiled and curled his mustache and knew the diagnosis now.

He took a little probe, called a doppler, and placed it on an artery as Tony listened in amazement to the high-pitched beeping sound of a normal artery. When the probe was placed over the artery of his thigh there was hardly a sound.

"There are several more tests I have to do, Tony. We want

you to sleep in our laboratory, and we are going to measure the ability of your penis to get hard during sleep."

Tony was placed in a comfortable, quiet room. A rubber-like balloon was placed around his penis, which would record any erections that occurred at night. This would be a test to determine if Tony's impotence was due to psychiatric causes or was organic. The doctor explained to Tony that there are periods of rapid eye movement during sleep, called vertical and horizontal, associated with certain brain-wave patterns. The penis responds by various degrees of erection. Four or five periods of rapid eye movements (REMs) have been recorded, and there is a close relationship between these eye movements and the swelling of the penis. In psychogenic impotence, sleep erections are normal, while if there is a medical organic reason, the erection that occurs in sleep are decreased or absent.

A piece of gauze was attached to Tony's penis with a monitoring device. If the piece of gauze stretches, it is recorded like an electrocardiogram, which is then read by the doctor the following morning.

The following morning, when the doctor arrived at Tony's room, there was no recording at all of an erection having occurred at night. He then ordered an arteriogram, an X ray of the arteries of the legs and abdomen, that confirmed his suspicion. At the point where the aorta of the abdomen divides into its branches for the legs, there was an obstruction: just a little amount of blood trickled down to the legs, and probably even less arrived at the penis. The diagnosis is called the Leriche syndrome.

This tale has a happy ending. A surgeon removed the obstruction in the artery, placed a graft, and Little Tony became the Stallion again.

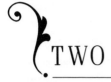

TWO

Dead Mackerel

AN ELEGANT WOMAN named Madeline lived in the village of R——; she was a wealthy stockbroker's wife known for her charity, intelligence, and her immaculate appearance. Each hair was in its place and she wore the latest fashions of the day. She was chairlady of the Board of Education, the local symphony, and she headed charity drives for the unfortunate. Everyone admired her charm. She was a devoted wife and mother and an excellent tennis player. There were no flaws in her character—no secret, unconscionable, bad thoughts in her brain. A walking Madonna, the ladies of the local DAR called her.

"She's too good to be true. There has to be something out of place," one of her crowd whispered maliciously.

She treated the nefarious-looking garbage collector as if he were the president of the bank. She shared all her good fortune with others, much to the chagrin of her husband who felt her generosity would ruin them. Not one molecule of her body held a speck of ill will, although she did have one weakness: She despised fish. Since childhood, she feared the sight and smell of the slimy Pisces. No one knew of this phobia—not her mother, not her father, not her husband, not her children. Never in her house was one of the sea served on her plate.

Once at a splendid dinner party when fish was served, she was filled with repulsion. Politely, with a white silken hand, she pushed the Dover sole away from her sight. "I break out in hives and my throat closes," she automatically told the hostess who quickly replaced it with a chicken leg.

Apart from her fish problem she was on top of the world until, one day, her stockbroker husband dropped dead of a heart attack while playing golf, and her world collapsed.

There were many eligible bachelors waiting in the wings who wanted to marry her, but no one could replace her Elmer.

"Sell the house," her married daughter said, "and you can come and live with us." She would not hear of it and remained in mourning indefinitely.

Elmer's study remained untouched. His clothing still hung in the closet; even his robe stayed over the chair in the bedroom. Months passed and she never appeared at any of the board meetings or the town symphony; she refused dinner engagements and stopped playing tennis. She became a recluse. Her housekeeper was discharged and she subsisted on frozen foods and vegetables and sat home all day watching television.

When she was seen by her old friends, they could barely recognize her. Her once-coiffured hair now looked like Medusa's head. She became fat from eating chocolate cookies. Her eyes were always swollen because she cried and moaned each day as she spoke to Elmer, especially at four o'clock in the afternoon, their cocktail hour. Elmer was with her in thought every minute of the day.

The oldest daughter tried everything to bring her mother

around, but no words could dissuade her. Her daughter brought in food because she refused to leave the house, and saw to it that the sheets were changed and the clothing was laundered.

Many months later, one night before going to bed, Madeline thought she smelled fish on her body, a repugnant stench. She surmised that her daughter had had the temerity to bring stale fish into the house. She dug into the refrigerator, searching frantically for rotten fish. She removed the pies, the peas, the porridge, the frozen pizzas, TV dinners, a dozen eggs, a container of milk, and cream cheese and threw them into the garbage. With vengeance, through the early hours of the morning, she scrupulously scrubbed the refrigerator until it gleamed. Then, on her knees, she washed the tiles in the kitchen with a fury. Exhausted and drenched in sweat, she fell asleep on top of her bed.

Morning came, and the smell of fish still lingered. She stripped off her nightgown, pushed it in the laundry bag outside the door for her daughter, then went into a spacious marble bathroom and showered. She scrubbed her body mercilessly with a handbrush until each inch of skin was as red as a lobster. The Opium perfume, Elmer's favorite, she generously spread all over her body, and moaned, "Will not the perfumes of Arabia clean this lily white hand?" She tried to quote Lady Macbeth in her despair.

She screamed out to her daughter. "How dare you buy stale fish and put it somewhere! Rotten food that causes my body inside to rot. That's it!" she yelled. Her organs inside were rotting away like a cadaver eaten by maggots. Maggots eating her spleen, her kidneys, her lungs. "Something is rotten in Denmark!" she yelled.

She ran to her wardrobe closet and pulled out the dresses she now never wore. After one hour she looked into the mirror and saw her old self: her hair neatly combed, her makeup expertly placed, and the beautiful French designer dress that had shoulders like a football player. For the first time in four months, she went out in the street. The air was fresh and breezy and there was no longer that inexorable smell. She walked for hours, feeling relieved, as if a great burden had been lifted from her body.

On the way home she stopped to visit her daughter. Once in her daughter's house, the smell returned—the stale smell of rotten fish.

"I smell a fish," she told the daughter. "It's terrible! I'm not going crazy."

The daughter went close to her mother and smelled the Opium perfume on her body but not the fish.

The doctor who examined her was thorough and ordered many tests, but found no illness.

"I think your mother is psycho, and we had better send her to a shrink."

Dr. L., on Madison Avenue, a renowned psychiatrist, showed Madeline pictures with black spots and asked her what she saw. Her reply, "Dead mackerels."

His diagnosis was clear. Madeline was suffering from a serious psychosis, depression, and schizophrenia, which had been triggered off by the death of her husband. Medication was prescribed, psychiatric sessions were arranged, but Madeline continued to become worse and she held fast to her complaint.

Her obsession became so great that when her daughter took her to a restaurant, she swooned when the waiter trudged by with a fried trout on his serving tray. She no longer was a recluse, because the only relief she received was to walk the streets like a trollop for endless hours into the night, until, too exhausted to go on, she returned home to sleep.

While each session with the psychiatrist was always the same, turning over and over her obsession with the smell, the psychiatrist began to think he smelled rotten fish on her body. He had known cases of patients who were called hyperosmic—an undue sensitivity to odors—a prominent symptom of schizophrenia. Yet, after she left, there was a faint odor of a dead swordfish that lingered in his small office. He sniffed the air, the walls, the chair where Madeline sat. There was a slight tinge of decay. He had learned in his training how some doctors contracted their patient's illnesses. Had he become victim to this folie?

In a panic haste, before his next consultation, he took his lemon air spray and inundated his office. He covered the chair, his desk, and the mouthpiece of his telephone. When the room smelled of a tropical garden, he was satisfied and saw the next patient.

Frustrated and convinced that she was suffering from a strange illness, Madeline decided to check into a large medical center and was given a private room. Several days later, in the morning when the professor arrived to visit her, he told the interns that the room smelled like a dead mackerel.

The professor, whose nose was supersensitive, examined her body carefully and found that her forehead was covered with thick vertical folds of skin hidden by her makeup. The skin of her face and arms was slightly elastic and dry and there were some excoriations on her arms. Her skin was scaly—like a carp.

A routine blood count was normal, as well as a chest X ray and liver tests, and dozens of others. The professor, a renowned maven on difficult diagnoses, scratched his shiny head.

Question: What smells like fish but isn't fish? No answer came to him. He searched frantically through textbooks of pharmacology on odors generated by chemical breakdowns in the body. Rotten egg smells came from hydrogen sulphur, by-products of protein. Then there it was, TMA: trimethylamine smells like a fish.

A tube was placed into her urinary bladder to collect the

urine, and by a special technique called gas chromatographic analysis, the TMA analysis was performed. This compound, normally not detectable in urine specimens, was found in abundance in her sample.

The professor explained to his students that the biochemical basis for the fish-odor syndrome may suddenly develop for no reason. The gut bacteria convert substances such as fish, eggs, liver, and kidney into TMA, which normally is destroyed by the liver unless there is a rare metabolic defect.

Madeline was placed on a diet devoid of fish, eggs, liver, and kidney, and there was an immediate lessening and a decrease in the frequency of the odor. But before the attacks were completely eliminated, she had to undergo a two-week course of a medicine called metronidazole hydrochloride, one pill three times a day. Her diet was restricted of soy beans, peas, mayonnaise, fish, eggs, liver, and kidney.

The chemical known as choline, which is found in eggs, is degraded by the gut bacteria to form TMA. Madeline had a defective enzyme system in which the TMA could not be further broken down and became excreted in the urine, in the breath, in the skin, and in the feces, and gave off the smell of fish.

To prove that he was correct, the professor administered again all the foods that she was forbidden and the odor reappeared. He also gave her some choline pills which again resulted in the fish odor reappearing because it had caused an elevation of TMA in the urine.

Madeline is now fully cured. She remarried to a lawyer, and although she never again smelled like a dead mackerel, she still has an aversion to fish.

THREE

The Kosher Connection

THE BROOKLYN JEWISH Hospital was located near the center of Hasidic life in the Crown Heights section of Brooklyn. The clinics and emergency rooms were usually crowded with men wearing their somber Hasidic garb of black frocks and fur hats, children with long ringlets, and observant women with their wonderfully colorful head shawls and faces untouched by cosmetics. Part of my internship training at this hospital, in 1963, was to spend six weeks in the medical clinic, a pleasant reprieve from the enervating schedule of working 36 hours nonstop on the medical ward and then having 24 hours to "recuperate."

My wife and I lived in a cockroach haven, a rat-infested apartment within walking distance of the hospital, and on a monthly stipend of sixty dollars, we were forced to eat all our meals in the hospital cafeteria, as did almost all the other interns and residents.

One morning in early March, I met Sarah and Augie at the medical clinic. Sarah, an Orthodox Jewess, 62 years old, with a cheerful round red face, was wearing a babushka covering her shaved head (a practice both of piety and practicality, the bald head "protecting" her from all but her husband). Her friend Augie, 70 years old, was the Italian shoemaker on the block; he had a generous and streetwise face and thick knobby hands from cutting leather and nailing shoes for forty years. Sarah came to the clinic each week to have her blood pressure and blood sugar level checked because she suffered from serious diabetes and needed large dosages of insulin to control her condition.

As I read through the chart, both Augie and Sarah sat quietly in front of my desk, a startling study of contrasts. It was evident that Sarah was fifty pounds overweight and paid little, if any, heed to medical advice. Her diabetes was consistently under poor control; yet she came to the clinic regularly—as if the visits themselves were enough to keep her well. To this day I am mystified about why some patients never miss a medical appointment but never do what they are told, their medical conditions deteriorating right in front of the physicians' eyes. No cajoling or prophecy of impending doom seems to change this. But I suppose I am no different. My periodontist lectures me about flossing each day, which I rarly do; yet I see him regularly for my periodontal checkup and listen to him with great fear as he warns me that my teeth will fall out when the gums surrender. For a week or so his words ring in my ear and I follow his orders, then the ringing grows distant and finally disappers.

"My chart is as fat as I am," she said. "You are the new doctor for the month. You look like such a nice doctor; you have such pretty eyes ['schayne aygen,' she said in Yiddish]. You're married? If not, I have such a beautiful girl for you, just right for your size. She is rich, too." She continued in this manner for another ten minutes, constantly pulling at her dress sleeves because they were as tight around her fat arms as a tourniquet. She wore thick-lensed glasses that magnified her eyes into two huge glass marbles. Her chart indicated that she had cataract operations and was now fitted with special glasses because of choroid degeneration, which had reduced her vision by fifty percent.

"How are you feeling, Sarah?" I finally asked, attempting to bring her back to the reasons that had brought her to the clinic. (It is no easy matter to be confronted with rambling patients and to tactfully return them to the central issues.)

"How do I feel, he asks?" and she looked at Augie. "If I felt all right, would I be here? What do you think? My head hurts all the time, my stomach aches, my feet are swollen, my muscles hurt, and I am all the time tired. Passover is coming, and I can't do my work. Do you know how much work I have to do for those good-for-nothings to make passover? Every dish has to be changed, every corner of the house has to be scrubbed, all the bread crumbs have to be removed. My husband, may he rest in peace, left me with a bunch of ungrateful children—such lazy bums!—but I am not here for me. I brought the goy with me." And she pointed to Augie who sat quietly smiling. She softly took one of Augie's knobby hands and proffered it to me like an offering.

"Look at these hands. They are swollen like mushrooms growing on them. He is in pain all the time and he can't work and he can't walk-at all; he walks like a chicken on the street."

His hands were deformed and the knuckles were red and bumpy. Behind my desk was a small examining table where I examined his other joints which had the classical signs of gouty arthritis. I told Sarah the good news that gout is one form of arthritis that can readily be treated and, in time, the medication can actually lessen or even make the ugly bumps of gout disappear.

"I knew it!' Sarah said, "Dr. Pretty Eyes will help you. Check my blood pressure, young doctor. I'm getting a headache." Her blood pressure was very high.

"Have you been taking your pills?" I asked.

"Of course. Every day, like they told me."

Augie quickly interjected, "She takes them when she feels like it. Not too often, sometimes less."

"Sarah, you must take the pills because if your blood pressure stays up so high you can get a stroke." She must have heard this admonition hundreds of times.

Her blood sugar was more than dangerously high. "Every day, I inject myself with 40 units of insulin before breakfast like they taught me, right in the thigh." Unabashedly, she raised her huge flowered dress, exhibiting a fat scarred thigh. "My pin cushion has less holes than me."

Sarah was taking her insulin, but I discovered that, because of her poor vision, she was unable to draw the correct number of units into the insulin syringe. After the clinical nurses provided her with a special syringe with the units printed in large bold letters, her blood sugar decreased, although it still remained dangerously high.

With each visit Sarah brought home-baked cakes, which she distributed to the nurses and aides like calling cards, and Augie brought homemade wine, which he gave to interns in small dark bottles. Together, they looked like an old Slavic painting of peasants as they entered through the revolving clinic door— Sarah, small, round, red of face, the richly-colored scarf around her head; and Augie, dark, wearing a rumpled black suit, white shirt, black tie, and a black hat, holding Sarah's hand, smiling, showing a full set of wonderfully white teeth against his dark complexion.

"He is a miracle man," Sarah yelled. "He was a cripple, this goy." Her shrill voice was heard throughout the clinic. Augie's arthritis had improved greatly with the medications for gout, one chronic illness that often reacts so quickly and positively to the proper medications that it makes the doctor seem like an inspired healer.

"Pretty Eyes, I brought you a cheesecake for you and your wife. Augie, give him the wine. The doctor looks anemic. Next week is Passover, Doctor. You come with your wife to my Seder."

The clinic staff had drawn lots for the holidays. I had drawn Christmas and was free on Passover, and I gratefully accepted her generous invitation.

At sunset, we arrived at Sarah's two-family house in Crown Heights, in the heart of the Hasidic neighborhood. The family was seated around a very long oak table which was covered with a brilliantly white, embroidered tablecloth and held twelve large candlesticks and gleaming plates and silverware. The scene could have been used for an idyllic Passover setting for a wall painting. Everything was suffused with the festive odors of Passover—gefilte fish, soup, chicken, condiments, wine, fruit. The oldest son was resplendent in a white ceremonial frock, leaning on a huge and fluffy pillow, holding a silver prayer book. The men wore prayer shawls around their shoulders and hats, and the women sat together at the end of the table with the children. But there was no sign of Augie. After the first set of prayers were said, the youngest one of the crowd, five years old, recited the four Passover questions: "Why is this night different from all other nights?" and then for the rest of the long and lovely evening the responses were given, a short and dramatic history of the exodus of the Jews from Egypt.

Sarah appeared to be weary, a sick expression was on her face, as if she smelled something wrong. She lacked her usual vigor, her gregariousness; the mischevious twinkle in her eyes was absent.

"Your husband has to save me like he did for Augie, you know. I feel terrible. All my muscles hurt, but I shouldn't be talking like this at the Seder," she said to my wife.

"Where is Augie?" I asked Sarah.

"Downstairs in his apartment, where he always is." I wasn't going to ask more because she seemed annoyed.

By nine o'clock we hadn't even started to eat, but we had drunk plenty of kosher wine. Sarah's face had become scarlet red and she rarely sat down at the table she had so laboriously prepared. She was too busy serving everyone else, although she managed to sit and sip her wine at the appropriate blessings. I knew the havoc the wine was going to play on her diabetes, but I dared not say a word. Intuitively she caught my eye, silently saying, "I know all this will make me suffer later, but Passover comes once a year. I am not like that goy downstairs who sits all day drinking his dandelion wine."

Attending a patient's dinner is always an uneasy experience, especially if there is a specific diet involved. You watch them eat, and you enjoy a sumptuous meal that often includes, in heaping measure, everything they are forbidden to eat.

"Tonight we are making an exception, right Doctor? Tomorrow I will start my diet, I promise." The eternal promise of the overweight patient, the chronic alcoholic, or the heavy cigarette smoker: *"Tomorrow,* I will be good." Most of the time, tomorrow never comes, or, if it does, it is too late. I suddenly realized that probably more than 80 percent of the illnesses I treat are caused by the wrong things patients do, and I wondered if there is some side of self-destruction in all of us.

Sarah again disappeared into the kitchen, reappearing minutes later, struggling with a mammoth engraved silver platter carrying her famous gefilte fish. She spun it around for everyone to see and just barely had the strength to set it down. She huffed and puffed like a steam engine and said, "Eat! Everyone eat!" Who could ignore such a command? It was the most delicious gefilte fish I ever ate. Actually, this was the first large formal Seder I had attended since I was in Europe in 1939, in the city of Danzig, where I was born. This Seder was so similar to that one that for a moment I was transported back almost thirty years to when I was a child, the same night when the Nazi's destroyed the synagogue next to our house and we were arrested and sent to Gestapo headquarters. (We miraculously escaped one month before the onset of World War II.)

"You are daydreaming, Pretty Eyes," I heard Sarah say. "Do you like my gefilte fish?"

"It is exquisite."

"Then you will come every year from now on, God willing, if I am still alive."

After the fish came the chicken soup with the delicate knaydlech, those round luscious matzo balls, and the chicken. One dish followed the other, endlessly interrupted with prayers and singing; finally, the front door was opened to allow the spirit of Elijah the Prophet to enter to bless the table. (A full glass of wine awaited him. As children we could swear he drank it.)

At the conclusion of the Seder I asked Sarah why Augie was not present. Perhaps he was not well, or maybe they had had a squabble.

"Goyim are not allowed at the Seder. I have to keep the tradition for my family. Don't worry, he will get the whole meal. He finished the gefilte fish already with his buddies from his Italian club. Tell him not to smoke those disgusting black stokers. They smell up his bedroom."

"How long have you known Augie?" I asked.

"That wop? Since we were children. He lived downstairs with his mother."

"Did you ever want to marry Augie?"

"What a question! An Orthodox Jew marrying a goy? My father would have thrown me out of the house. My marriage was already arranged before I even knew Augie. My husband was a good man, but dull and stupid. He gave me three nasty sons," she whispered. "He suddenly died and left me a small insurance policy to live on."

As she was talking I observed that Sarah's face was swollen; it was not just fat. Some diabetics develop kidney failure and the body swells up like a whale; perhaps this dreaded complication had set in. I dared not say anything to Sarah at the Seder.

"Why are you staring at my face? I know it is swollen."

"It is somewhat, Sarah," I said.

"On Monday I will let you examine me," she said.

At two in the morning the Seder ended. Her sons had barely talked to me. They regarded me as a philistine even though I had a strong education in Jewish tradition and read Hebrew.

Three days later, on Sunday morning, Augie called me at home, which he often did to invite me and my wife for wine and cheese. (Augie made the wine from dandelions from the backyard of the house, and distilled them in old kegs that had belonged to his father.)

"Doctor," he said, "Sarah is in the ER. I think she had a stroke this morning." His voice sounded grief stricken, trembling with pain.

Lounging in bed Sunday morning and then having a leisurely breakfast and reading the *Times* was, unfortunately, not part of a doctor's life; ten thousand not unsimilar interruptions lay ahead in my medical career.

It was hardly surprising that Sarah had had a stroke. Her blood pressure was always poorly controlled, she was a diabetic, and she was 62 years old; it was not likely she would be spared. There is a saying among some in the medical profession that only nice people get the bad diseases, and Sarah seemed to fit the description only too well.

When I arrived at the ER, Augie was sitting in the waiting room, looking gray and stooped, his knobby hands dangling lifelessly between his legs. The neurologist had already performed his examination. Sarah was in a semi-coma, barely breathing, and she was paralyzed; her temperature was 104 degrees.

"She is my patient in the clinic," I told the attending neurologist.

"It may not be a stroke," the neurologist said. "It could be meningitis."

In 1960s we did not have such sophisticated tests as a CAT scan to diagnose the cause of coma. I assisted the resident in performing a spinal tap to see if it contained blood—a major undertaking because she was so obese. The fluid was clear, but it did show infectious cells, which made the diagnosis of meningitis seem accurate. Both strokes and meningitis can cause coma and paralysis.

Augie was anxiously waiting for me to tell him the news.

"I told her every day to stop eating all the cakes and to take her pills. She would not listen," he cried. "It is my fault. I should have tried harder."

"We all should have, Augie." Even to this day, when one of my patients suddenly does badly, I feel I should have tried harder.

"You see Doctor, she never believed she was sick. She trusted none of the other doctors. She planned after Passover to lose weight and surprise you. I don't think it was her diabetes that made her so sick. It is something else. I know this woman. She has been acting funny for at least a week. She always complained of everything hurting her, except this time it was always her muscles and her back and her head. Sarah is a very strong woman, a good woman. Nothing was ever too much for her. It took all her strength to get the Seder ready. Not one of those bum children of hers helped. They pray all day and run a little religious shop that gives them some money."

"You help Sarah with money, too?"

"Just a little. I have plenty. More than I need for my old age. If she needs any specialists, I have enough to pay for them. Watch how all her bum sons come running now because they know she has a little money stashed away, and they want to be sure they get their hands on it. They're afraid I will get it."

As he finished talking, the three sons arrived, wearing their traditional garb, and were angry with the neurologist. Since then I have learned that many families who are guilt-ridden blame the doctors, the nurses, and the condition of the hospital for a bad result. They blamed me for allowing her blood pressure and diabetes to be so poorly controlled. They decided that Sarah had become ill because she had received poor medical attention. Today, most probably, a lawyer would have already been consulted, a malpractice suit initiated.

Augie stayed with Sarah night and day, sitting at her bedside, holding her hand, whispering to her like a teenage lover. He was certain she heard every word in her semi-stuporous state. Every day he brought fresh flowers cut from his garden, and his gentle voice read the papers to her like a child just learning to read. Each day Sarah began to improve on her own, and the sons' visits became less frequent.

Augie wanted her to have a private room and her own doctor, but as she began to regain her ability to speak she made it clear that she trusted only the hospital doctors and that a private room was extravagant.

"Better save your money for old age, Augie. You may be next."

Although her meningitis improved, she still looked sickly. Her eyelids and face remained swollen; she developed purple spots on her arms and legs that looked like crawling spiders. She could not get out of bed because her muscles were too painful. The neurologist diagnosed her to have a muscle disorder, probably of viral origin, which had also caused her meningitis. Arthritis experts suggested that her illness was an infection of the arteries and muscles called vasculitis, a deadly disease.

Sarah thought she was suffering from cancer and that the doctors were lying to her. "Tell me, Pretty Eyes, what do I got? Those dummies don't know anything. You have to save me. Augie can't manage without me. If I have cancer, tell me."

How often do elderly patients think doctors hide things from them, especially when things are not going well! Cancer was always foremost in the mind; more recently, people also fear they are suffering from AIDS when obscure symptoms appear.

"Sarah, those so-called dummies are the best doctors in the hospital, and they are experts."

There is no other time in the life of a doctor when he is more knowledgeable than as an intern. His training in medical school has been completed and he is studying for the national licensure boards. The knowledge is there but not the clinical experience or the seasoned intuition of an older practitioner. So when the blood tests showed a high eosinophil count in the blood, I researched all the causes for a high count in the medical library. Interns have a penchant for ordering too many blood tests to make certain nothing is missing, and I was no exception. One of the tests I did order, which was an unlikely diagnosis for a kosher woman like Sarah, was the blood test for trichinosis. A shot in the dark. It was like ordering a test for syphilis on a nun.

Trichinosis is a parasitic disease which often resulted from eating pork. According to Jewish dietary law, eating pork is strictly prohibited because pork is considered unclean, a source of illness. Pure sanitary expediency. The wise rabbis were also good doctors.

The following day the test for trichinosis returned—positive! But how was it possible?

Sarah became more and more alert, but her eyelids and face remained swollen and all her muscles were painful. She developed a rash on her body that looked like measles. The neurologist decided the diagnosis was polymyositis or Hodgkin's disease. But when the titer for trichinosis returned, rising higher each day, all the consultants agreed she was really suffering from trichinosis. They all congratulated me for my astuteness, knowing full well it was a lucky guess. (With maturity, diagnosing a rare disease often becomes an *educated* guess.)

Since I arrived at the diagnosis by pure chance, it was my responsibility to tell Sarah the diagnosis, which was, to say the least, a sensitive issue. I met Augie in the waiting room and asked him, "Augie, do you ever cook for Sarah?"

"Once in ten years. She won't eat on my dishes because I am not kosher."

"Augie, is it possible that Sarah has eaten some pork in the past few months?"

"Never! Sarah would rather die than eat pork."

"Well, Augie, she must have had some pork because she is suffering from an illness that you can only catch from eating unkosher meat—rabbits, pork, boar," and I continued with a list I had just memorized in the library. "I will have to tell her, you know."

"You can tell her, and she won't believe you or any of the other doctors; then she really will think she has cancer."

The following morning, Sarah was receiving the medication for trichinosis, and if the diagnosis was correct, all her muscle weakness would disappear and the poliomyelitis-like clinical picture would be gone. Augie was right. Sarah only laughed when I told her the diagnosis and called us all *"naren,"* one of her favorite words—"fools."

"If you cooked food that was contaminated with pork," I said to her, "you are not to blame. You couldn't be blamed for breaking the law."

"I go to the best kosher butcher in the neighborhood. You disappoint me, Doctor, and I thought you had some brains. Pretty eyes, but no common sense. How could a kosher butcher carry pork? A kosher butcher located in a Hassidic area?"

I asked Sarah how it was possible for an Orthodox Jew to spend almost all her time with an Italian Catholic.

"Now you are being fresh, but you do make your point. Maybe I will be written up in Ripley's 'Believe It or Not.'"

A real "fascinoma," the hospital staff called it. Soon all the fourth-year medical students and interns came to talk to Sarah, who enjoyed the attention, but she refused to be examined until she was showered, her lipstick was on, and her bed sheets were changed. On Saturday morning, when all the interesting cases were presented, Sarah drew a packed house. This was my first presentation of a patient history and discussion in front of one hundred people. All my review articles were organized, and the night before I recited the story of Sarah to my wife—an actor rehearsing his part. The title of the conference was "The Kosher Connection." The conference went well, but no one had a plausible explanation about how the culprit had entered into Sarah's kosher system. Perhaps this was the making of a new disease, a new clinical entity—Jewish trichinosis.

Every kosher butcher has to be certified by the rabbi, just as all kosher products have to be tested for purity. Somehow, Sarah had ingested the larvae of trichinosis without knowing it. I returned to Sarah to find the answers.

"I buy only the best, cleanest food," she said, "in kosher places. I never eat in restaurants or gentile homes."

"How do you make gefilte fish?" I asked her.

"Like I have been doing all my life, and my mother before."

"Well, tell me in detail."

"That is my own recipe, a family secret."

"I promise Sarah, it will be regarded as professional secrecy. I won't tell anyone." Sarah remained silent, moving her lips as if she were talking to someone not in the room. She was debating with herself about what to do. Sarah was also known to consult her dead mother when faced with a dilemma. "What would *she* do?"

"All right, I see no harm. You won't remember it, anyway." (How wrong she was; I still use her secret formula every year!)

"I buy pike fish. Most of the other women buy carp or another kind of white fish."

"Where do you buy it?" I asked.

"In the kosher store, of course. The *ganif* ("crook") then filets it for me and cleans it. I take it home, put it in the refrigerator, and then grind it myself. I add salt, pepper, and a slice of onion, a carrot, and a dozen of eggs; I add some more salt and pepper, and, of course, I taste it to see if it's seasoned just right; then I add a little garlic and parsley and just a touch of wine and mustard. Then comes the matzo meal—you have to have matzo meal—and then you boil the water, and then you have gefilte fish."

"That is all there is to it?" I asked teasingly. "Sarah, do you always taste the fish before cooking it?"

"Of course. After I boil it for two-and-a-half hours, it is too late, no?"

In the next two weeks, Sarah began to improve progressively, which made Augie very happy. He continued to come each day, bringing flowers and reading the *Brooklyn Eagle* to her. He had to begin with the obituary column. "At our age," Sarah said, "they drop like flies." And then followed the baseball news because Sarah was an ardent Dodger fan who had never seen a baseball game in her life but had fallen in love with Jackie Robinson.

Augie also brought in food hidden under the newspaper. For many weeks, we couldn't understand why her blood sugar and her blood pressure kept rising, until one evening I saw her eating a salami sandwich. A rather common and frustrating problem in hospitals.

"She insisted I bring her food," Augie said, "otherwise she would not let me come."

"How can I eat this pig food of the hospital," she said. "Then I really will die."

As soon as we put an end to the care packages that Augie brought, her diabetes came under control, as did her blood pressure.

On my day off several weeks later, I decided to walk towards the Brooklyn museum. I passed the kosher store where Sarah bought her fish and meat. Was it intuition, curiosity, whatever? I found myself standing inside the store where the proprietor was chopping meat with a cleaver. I was the only patron in the store and innocently asked the butcher if I could have some pork chops. I expected to be driven out like some maniac intruder, or to have the cruel meat cleaver flung at my head. Instead, the bearded man placed several pork chops on a butcher's block, the same block he used to filet the carp for gefilte fish.

With great difficulty, I had the pork chops inspected by the Department of Health, and they found the meat he carried was infested with the cysts of trichinosis. The parasite had infiltrated the fish from the butcher's block. Since Sarah tasted the raw fish, she had many times become infected with the larvae. The kosher butcher was not so kosher. The folks of the Hasidic community were up in arms. It had also become apparent that other innocent customers had been suffering from trichinosis. The butcher was no longer certified by the rabbi and lost all his kosher clientele.

While most cases of trichinosis improve without any treatment, some, rarely, like Sarah, become severely ill and may even die if not treated.

Sarah made a complete recovery, and years later I was heartbroken to learn that she had died of a stroke. Augie moved from New York to New Haven, where he became my very first patient when I started my practice. He died ten years later of cancer of the stomach.

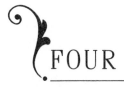

FOUR

The Blue Bloater

"DOCTOR, PLEASE SEE my husband. He is desperately ill." This call from the wife of one of my patients arrived in the late afternoon, on one of those hot and harried summer days.

"How long has he been ill?"

"Just a few weeks," she answered in a timorous voice. "He wanted to wait because he thought he would feel better."

"What's the problem?" My voice must have sounded angry because there was a momentary silence, then I heard her weeping, and her voice came on again.

"He can't breathe right. His face is blue. He sits on the chair choking for air."

"I think that you'd better take him right to the emergency room."

"He'll never go to the emergency room," she said. "He's afraid of hospitals. Please let me bring him to your office, I beg you."

"There's nothing I can do for him here."

His wife was pleading for his life as persistently as he had once ignored hers when she was critically ill in the intensive care unit. I vividly recalled how I had repeatedly tried to contact him, only to be informed by his office that he was out of town or busy with pressing matters.

An hour later, when most of my patients had left, I heard loud voices, and then a huge man entered my office accompanied by his two sons and his wife. He stood in the center of the room, his body bent into the letter C, gasping for air like a blowfish out of water, his face purple, his eyes red as fire. The few patients in the waiting room stared with fright as he slowly shuffled forward, each step accompanied with a pitiful gasp. When I came close to him, he raised his head and peered at me with desperate eyes.

"Take him into the examining room and get some oxygen!" I shouted to my nurses.

His sons and I struggled to set him on the examining table as his wife stood by, wringing her hands.

"Harry, it isn't so bad. The doctor isn't going to harm you. Just let him take care of you."

His arm was too large for the blood-pressure cuff. When I asked him some questions, he wasn't able to answer because he needed each breath to stay alive. I placed my stethoscope on his tattooed chest, knowing in advance that I would not be able to hear his heart, only the loud gurgling noises that sounded like a hot spurting geyser.

One of the nurses took the small cylinder of oxygen and attached the nasal prongs to his flaring nostrils. His face was now becoming darker, and his hands were as blue as the sea. Surely he would die at any moment, and there would be no hope to resuscitate him because his body—bloated and immense—would somehow have to be hefted to the floor, and the examining room was too small for such maneuvering.

"You'll have to go to the hospital," I said. "There is little I can do for you here."

He glared at me in anger, but his wife implored him, "Please dear, let the doctor call an ambulance. He will take care of you in the hospital—won't you, Doctor? You won't let anyone else touch him. And I'll stay with you all the time, and you'll see, in a few days, you'll be home."

His two sons—one 32 years old, the other 40—tall, erect, handsome, and neatly dressed, had no resemblence to the poor old man. They remained silent, staring off into space. Finally, one spoke.

"You gotta go, Dad. There's no other way."

I took his hand to reassure him, and finally he lowered his head and nodded up and down, like the fat lady at the circus.

So many times, for so many years, I have waited like that for the ambulance to arrive. At any moment the heart could stop. I often wondered if patients knew when they were so close to death. He didn't seem to know. He was too busy trying to breathe. Having a doctor so near, the oxygen prongs in his nose, the nurses at his side, must have given him reassurance. He took my hand into his, as if to hold onto life. How could he realize how helpless we were? Could he notice the pallor of my nurses, or hear my own heart pounding? Where was that ambulance that would set me free? I tried to busy and calm myself by again placing the stethoscope on his chest. Once more I listened to the turbulence within him.

The ambulance finally arrived. Two men and a young woman carried a stretcher. "Here, in this room," my receptionist told them.

The drivers saw the task before them. The room was too small to get him onto the stretcher. He would have to be lifted off the examining table and carried into the waiting room. The three attendants went on one side, the two sons and I on the other. His wife held his head like a gourd. We lifted almost half a ton of man.

"Did he have a heart attack, Doc?" one of the ambulance men asked.

"I don't know. I think his heart and lungs are bad."

Carrying the blue, puffing man, we struggled through the narrow corridor and at last reached the stretcher. He was carried off, a giant on a toothpick. As the door closed, his wife saw despair, and relief, in my eyes.

"Is he going to be all right, Doctor? Thank you so much for letting me bring him here. I know you'll take good care of him."

The remaining patients had left my office. There had been too much sickness there that day. The nurses silently returned to the malodorous room, removed the crumpled paper on the examining table, disposed of the small tank with its prongs, and sprayed disinfectant to clear the air. For them, the day was over.

Hours later when I arrived at the hospital, he was in the intensive care unit, lying in a special room; a tube in his throat was connected to a respirator. He sounded like a man breathing through a tunnel. His color was much less blue, but he still had that dusky death-like appearance. His wife sat next to the bed, studying the monitor as his heart lines raced across the screen, the pattern becoming irregular each time he moved his giant frame.

The man looked like he was sleeping in a busy railroad station, oblivious to the activity around him. It was early July. The unit was crowded with the new interns, residents, students, and young nurses. They seemed to look brighter and younger each year. I marveled about so many machines and people caring for one man. The new intern, Calvin, crisp in his white uniform, carried an air of confidence as the resident gave the instructions. The nurse that attended could have been the intern's sister. Her hair was straw-colored and her eyes were blue as she moved gently and confidently around the room, checking all the life-saving connections with great efficiency.

"His blood gases were terrible," the intern said, "so we intubated him. His heart had stopped when he arrived in the emergency room."

"He's very ill," I told his wife outside the room.

"I know you're doing everything."

"How long has he really been sick?"

She hesitated. "A while. A couple of weeks."

"Not so," one son said. "He's been ill for months."

"How would you know?" the other son said. "You haven't seen him in years."

Throughout the night, his wife sat at the bed. The nurse brought her a tray of food and told her it would be better for her to get some rest. Perhaps later the next day they would remove the throat tube.

The following morning, when I arrived at the hospital, the sick man's wife was still sitting in a large lounging chair, and for the first time, I noticed she was the counterpart of her husband. Her head was as round as a gourd; her mouth so wide that it looked artificial. She struggled to raise herself from the chair and began to smile nervously. Linda, the young nurse, continued with the care of the man, wiping the spittle from the tube that formed bubbles around his mouth, arranging his pillow, and checking the monitor, oblivious to my presence. She finally spoke.

"His heart became irregular. He was started on lidocaine last night."

His wife looked at me, waiting for an explanation.

"We use this medicine to regulate his heart." She glanced at the monitor as if she understood.

"He is doing better, Mrs. R. We'll probably remove the tube if the oxygen of his blood is good."

"What happened to him?" she asked in a very gentle tone.

"He is suffering from pneumonia and heart failure. He must've had a lung disease for a long time, and now he developed that kind of pneumonia called Legionnaire's disease. But with the antibiotics and other treatment he is receiving, we hope he will respond. We are doing everything possible."

"Oh, I know. I can see that. Everyone is so good to him, especially Linda. She is wonderful."

Linda was from Columbus, Ohio, and her husband was a first-year medical student at the university. Just looking at her could make anyone feel better. She rarely smiled, but when she did, the room glowed like bright sunshine.

At five o'clock in the afternoon of the third day, Linda had cut the tube while Calvin gently slipped it from his mouth. The patient was alert and breathed freely on his own.

His wife, with a relieved and gratified expression on her face, said, "Now I can go home and get some sleep." She took Linda's hand and kissed it. "I am so grateful to you and the doctor. I want to buy you a present."

"That isn't necessary."

"Please let me do this."

After his wife left, Linda finished cleaning the respiratory equipment and checked the I.V. in his arm.

"Hang in there, Harry. Keep doing so well, and you soon will be home."

He gave her a strange hesitant smile, and with a froggy voice, he tried to speak. It sounded garbled, as if coming from a record placed on the wrong speed, and the language was incomprehensible. As he spoke louder, he mixed his words with vulgarities, rubbish, and then he started to growl.

"What can I do for you, Harry? Everything is all right."

With his head, he beckoned to the chair where a pair of crumpled pants were lying.

"Oh, you want your pants." She broke out in a radiant smile, almost laughing. "Of course." Linda walked around the other side of the bed, picked up his pants, as roomy and baggy as a potato sack, and then draped them across his protruding belly.

"What can I get you from your pants? What do you have that's so important?" She began to giggle.

His eye stopped roaming and his mouth gaped open as his right hand suddenly tugged at the I.V., tearing it out of his wrist. He jerked the other arm loose and both arms become drenched in blood.

"Harry, stop that immediately!" She looked toward the outside of the cubicle for help. The secretary at the desk had her back turned.

"Hey, get somebody in here quick!"

The blue-faced man pulled the belt from his pants as Linda tried to restrain his muscular arms and push him back into bed. "You have to stay in bed! You are too strong for me. Now be a good boy, Harry."

Cursing and growling, he pitched his body up like a whale about to surface and lassoed the belt around her neck. Linda struggled to release the belt, her screams smothered as he tightened the hold. Calvin ran into the room and pulled the large arms with all his strength as Linda turned blue. Other doctors and nurses arrived and grabbed his arms. They thrust needles into his veins, punched him in the face, tugged and pulled and struggled until, at last, he was subdued.

Linda was bruised and in a state of shock. Her color returned quickly to pink. "My God, he was going to kill me!"

When I arrived later, his wife was sitting on a couch in the waiting room with a nurse at her side, and a priest. She smiled her pumpkin smile when I entered the room.

"Is my husband bad? You must have bad news for me."

"Your husband's condition has changed for the worst, but he is alive . . ." and I hesitated for an instant, very conscious of the eyes of the priest on me.

I was filled with remorse and great pity for this woman. A few minutes earlier I had seen her husband lying in restraint, still growling and screaming, his face blue, his eyes bulging out of their sockets. The intravenous medication they had injected to subdue him had already worn off.

"Your husband, did he ever strike you?"

"Oh, no! He's the best man a woman could have. He was always kind to me, brought his paycheck to me each week. Naturally, we had our arguments. Doesn't everybody?"

"Your husband seems to have suddenly lost his mind. The lidocaine we gave him for his heart sometimes causes people to become disoriented and psychotic," I told her.

"I know he hates hospitals. He just wants to go home. Has he given anybody any trouble? I can talk to him. He will listen to me."

"Your husband has hurt one of our nurses."

The smile now left her face.

"He tried to strangle Linda with his belt."

"Oh, my God! Is she all right?"

"She is shaken, but she will be all right."

She remained silent. "It can't be," she said with a voice that came from the depths of her soul. "Harry wouldn't hurt anyone."

As we approached the sick man's room, two policemen were standing by the door and two of the hospital guards hovered over his bed. New sedation had started taking effect, and when his wife entered the room, she looked at him with a pitiful despairing glance, tears in her eyes. His heart was now beating erratically, and his face was bluer than ever as she touched his bruised cheek.

"He didn't know what he was doing," she whimpered. "Oh God, forgive him." He looked at her with a distant gaze.

"You aren't going to let him die?" she asked as the priest took her outside. While the interns were passing a tube back into his throat his heart suddenly stopped beating. As the alarm screeched, Calvin, the medical intern, pounded on his chest while the other resident climbed on the bed and pressed down on his chest. In a few seconds, the heart was beating again as the medication flowed into his body.

In the days that followed, Harry's condition improved somewhat. His heart rhythm remained normal. His lungs wheezed like a wooden stove. But he remained blue as before, and the oxygen level did not rise in his blood.

We kept Harry in the ICU because he remained cyanotic, but there was no explanation for it. His lung function tests did not reveal any abnormality that could account for the low oxygen, and various tests on his heart and circulatory system showed no blockages. We continued to administer oxygen to Harry in higher and higher concentrations, but the cyanosis persisted. We kept Harry in arm and body restraints, like a wild animal, and guards were constantly nearby.

"Do you have to keep Harry like this," his wife bemoaned each day to the staff. "Let me take him home. I can take care of him, and his sons will help." But she knew that once Harry went home it would only be she who would care for him.

The hospital psychiatrist was called in to assess Harry's mental state. If he was criminally insane, he would have to be committed, but as long as he remained blue it would not be possible to transfer him to a mental institution, and 24-hour hospital supervision and the body restraints would have to be continued. The interview took an hour. The psychiatrist met us in the conference room; there was Calvin, the chief resident, the floor nurse, and me. He read his report to us.

"Our blue-bloated friend is a retired truckdriver who was in the United States Army during World War II. In the past few months he lost his patience quickly, the smallest annoyances made him lose his temper. He struck his wife on several occasions. He does have marked paranoid tendencies and displays a great deal of hostility and anger towards authority, including his wife and sons, and now towards his doctors."

"What else is new?" the chief resident interjected.

"My conclusion is that he is a dangerous man and capable of aggressive acts because the low oxygen in his blood and the lidocaine he received has affected his brain. As long as you cannot correct his oxygen level, we will have to keep him on complete restraints." The lidocaine was discontinued.

The neurologist had also examined Harry and found him to have a normal examination, except that he was suffering from migraine headaches. Included in his tests was a CAT scan of the brain, as well as X rays of his arteries and other tests looking for blockages.

We were faced with a mega-dilemma of what to do for this blue man. Dozens of tests and consultants had not found the answer. Somewhere in the past, in the early days of my internship, I somehow recalled a similar case, but the details had now escaped me. One splendid professor from my medical school had once said, "If you want to know about your patients, visit their homes, learn about their lifestyle, see their surroundings, and you will be able to provide better care and find some answers."

The following day, I called Harry's wife and invited myself to her home. She lived in a two-family house in a middle-class neighborhood where all the houses looked the same.

Mrs. R. met me at the door, wearing a flowered housecoat.

"Please, Doctor, do come in. I have been baking some apple

cakes. Harry loves them. I thought I would bring an extra one for the staff."

The living room was tiny and neat, and in the center stood a small couch covered with flower-patterned plastic. It stood adjacent to a large easy chair that faced the television set. On small tables and on a dresser were dozens of artificial flowers. Mrs. R. saw me staring at them. "I make them. I have them all over the house. May I make some for you?"

"That would be very nice."

"Please sit down, Doctor. How about some coffee?"

She sat on Harry's chair and said, "Now there's got to be something very bad; otherwise, what other reason would you come here?"

"That is not so. Harry is doing as well as expected." I heard myself using the same old cliché. "We don't know why he is still blue and anemic. His lungs have improved and his heart is fine."

"But he was a terribly heavy smoker, Doctor. He always had a cigarette in his mouth, even when he was so sick."

"How bad were his migraine headaches? Did he become violent during his attacks?" I have known patients during their migraine headaches, when they become excruciatingly severe, to take lead pipes and strike themselves on their head. Sometimes they even attack others.

I had struck a sensitive chord because her eyes became moist. "Sometimes, but not very often. But he never really hurt me, and he always apologized and started crying."

"What sort of medications does he take when he gets his headaches?"

"He used to take pills that the doctor gave him, but now he buys them over the counter."

We went into the small bathroom and the medicine cabinet was packed with dozens of bottles of non-prescription medications, mostly aspirin and phenacetin-like combinations.

"Sometimes he takes ten, fifteen, or twenty, and I also put an icepack on his temples and massage the back of his neck. That helps."

We returned to the living room. "May I use your phone," I asked.

It was a wild hunch, so I called Calvin at the hospital and asked him to order a series of test for methemoglobinemia and sulfhemoglobinemia.

The following day the tests returned positive, which meant that the normal hemoglobin in Harry's blood had been replaced by a chemical that was unable to hold oxygen. Methemoglobinemia can cause cyanosis and bizarre behavior, just the kind Harry suffered from. It results when large amounts of aspirin or phenacetin-like compounds were taken for long periods of time in a susceptible person who may have a genetic abnormality of hemoglobin. Usually, once the medication is withheld the methemoglobinemia decomposes, the hemoglobin concentration returns to normal, the blueness disappears, and the anemia is corrected.

There still remained to be determined why, while in the hospital, he remained blue, anemic, and still had methemoglobinemia.

"Do you bring the pills to Harry at the hospital?" I asked his wife.

"Yes," she said. "Did I do something wrong? He asked me to because he was afraid he was not going to get them from the nurses."

The following day we substituted Vitamin C for the painkillers. Vitamin C tends to change the methemoglobinemia back to normal hemoglobin. In days to follow, the cyanosis disappeared; however, Harry's migraine headaches reappeared. Our neurologist at the hospital prescribed a program for him which controlled his headaches, and Harry was cautioned not to take medications that contained phenacetin.

He was discharged from the hospital, still suffering from chronic lung disease, but he gave up smoking and is living in Florida to this day.

FIVE

The Mad Hatter

Dr. S. was an outstanding dentist with an unblemished career of twenty-five years of practice. Not one patient ever drilled him with a complaint. Never did he invent a cavity or remove a crown before its time. He was also generous with his money, and an exemplary citizen who, for thirty years, was married to a woman every man could envy—sensitive, kind, intelligent, interesting, easy going, devoted to social welfare in the community. This blessed marriage produced two gifted children, a lawyer and a physician.

In this golden and glorious time of his life, the dentist began to think about retirement. Perhaps to the South; or maybe to work in a clinic in equatorial Africa at the Albert Schweitzer Hospital, sharing his skills with the less privileged. All options were open.

On the day before Christmas, something strange happened in his office. He was in a miserable mood and only grudgingly presented his receptionist and dental assistant with their bonuses. Totally out of character, he told them, "You don't deserve this Christmas bonus, not one dime, not one penny. You have been cheating me for years. I know what you have been doing—taking the cash and pocketing it and then giving false receipts to the patients." Both employees had been honest and faithful to the dentist for too many years to count and, naturally, were astounded by these terrible unfounded accusations. They had never seen him like that before.

He stormed out of the office, muttering blackly to himself and stopped at the local grocery store—for a Baby Ruth candy bar of all things.

This was equivalent to a rabbi buying a pound of bacon. Throughout his career, he had lectured his patients about the evils of sweets: "They will ruin your teeth!" he had warned, shaking his finger. And now he suddenly became a closet chocolate freak. Twelve Hershey bars, ten Mounds, chocolate Raisenettes, a dozen Baby Ruths—more, more, more. All of these he placed lovingly into his briefcase and smuggled into his house, even while his wife was cooking filet of sole in wine sauce and the delicate aroma of haute cuisine floated in the air.

His wife's gray hair was still radiant by candlelight as they sat at the table, which was lavishly set each night. She was used to his moods. He was entitled to be blue sometimes, especially after a hard day's work of drilling and filling and cleaning and shining so many teeth. Once he told her that he had cleaned over two hundred thousand teeth since he had started practicing. But his mood was deeper now. On this night, her husband sullen and silent, she knew better than to ask those most hairy questions: "What's the matter? Why are you so quiet?"

She had served his favorite dish, endives with olive oil and now waited expectantly for her husband to devour it. Instead, he just sat and barely nibbled on the Belgian delicacy. Then she served the filet of sole in a sauce of wine and nutmeg. He raised his fork, swallowed a piece with difficulty, pushed his plate aside. No longer could the good wife restrain herself. "Are you all right?"

The silence was smashed. "Of course I am all right. Stop nagging me, you bitch!"

Never in their thirty years of marriage had an unkind word or a vulgar sentence passed from the lips of this gentle soul. His wife, as if she had been struck by a sledgehammer, fell back in her chair, stunned.

"He must have had a really terrible day at the office," she thought. "I best say no more." She smiled quietly, but her silence did not scotch the insults which now shot across the table like a volley of cannonballs.

"You are a lazy woman!" he yelled. "Why don't you get a job like other women—like what do you call your friend?—Jane, the bitch!"

"Why don't you eat your fish, dear? It's good for you." Little did his wife know that his stomach was filled with crunch delights and Baby Ruths. There was no space for the sole, or anything.

The following day was Christmas, and it was snowing, as it should on Christmas day. All the dogwood and pine trees were covered with a white satin blanket. A Christmas tree towered majestically in the center of the spacious and gracious living room, rooted in lovely gift wrappings. The dentist had slept later than usual, and when he awoke his face was still covered by a cloud of sleep. He spoke not a word and dragged his weary body to the bathroom for his morning rituals.

When he saw the Christmas tree his face brightened, and then to his great dismay he realized that he had left his wife's present in the office. "I don't know what happened to me. I completely forgot this is Christmas, and I haven't been drinking," he told his wife in an apologetic voice, the very voice she was used to hearing all those good years. "My husband has returned," she told herself, "what a lovely gift."

It was a long weekend and friends came by with their greetings. They drank homemade eggnog laced with the finest brandy. Towards evening, like the sunset, the face of the dentist began to darken.

"I saw you outside with the delivery man," he told his wife.

"You did? And what did you see?" she said in a teasing voice.

"Don't be cute with me. You know you were kissing him. Kissing him right on the mouth, in front of everyone!" He continued his abusive charges until his wife, now in tears, placed her arms around his neck.

"My poor dear. Please stop. You are not well. Something is very wrong. Your staff tells me you are forgetting everything, that you placed a crown on the wrong tooth, fitted a prosthesis incorrectly. Please, dear, you must see a doctor. What has happened to you? I know you have been taking your phenobarbital for years. Are you taking more than you should?

As it turned out, the dentist was a phenobarbital addict. Long ago, when his revered father died, he had become a depressed, nervous wreck, and the family doctor had prescribed phenobarbital, which was then fashionable for anxiety. It made the doctor feel so good he kept refilling the open prescription for years. This was one of the more important secrets that he and his wife shared.

The following day the dentist flipped through the yellow pages and found my name. He checked with the medical society and discovered that I had just started my practice. Perhaps he liked this. Anyway, he arrived at my office looking like a dentist. He wore light summer pants and a jacket and hat that did not match, and golf shoes. It was Wednesday, the physician's day of rest, except for those early on in practice when every day is a day of rest—waiting for the patients to begin to arrive.

We sat in my new consultation office, lined with books and with furniture that shone like glass.

His wife, neatly coiffured and wearing a gray suit, sat by him, holding a pad and pencil and a list of notes. With so much time on my hands, I took a thorough history and then performed a two-hour physical examination. It was all of no avail. I had no explanation for his bizarre symptoms. Then, as they were about to leave my office, the wife said, "Oh, by the way, my husband takes phenobarbital for sleep."

The "Oh, by the way" is the most important sentence in medical practice. It is only then that the real reason for consulting a physician is often revealed. I teach my students to listen for this important sentence because a correct diagnosis may depend on just this.

I asked the dentist to return to my consulting room. It became clear that Dr. S. was addicted in the true sense of the word. Hardly surprising. Drug addiction was known to be frequent among healers, a reaction to uncommon stress.

During the next few months the dentist and I worked together to free him of his addiction. He stopped using phenobarbital, and seemed sometimes to be better, but all in all, he really did not improve. He was free of phenobarbital but perhaps it had been too long; perhaps the damage had already been done. Unfortunately, he continued to perform bad dentistry. Patients were leaving his practice, which began to dwindle, and he became more depressed.

Like a novice, he spent more time with each patient as his mental state worsened. Paranoia, depression, and memory loss were but a few of the obvious behavior aberrations he exhibited. I could do no more for him, and I suggested he seek psychiatric help.

Many months later, in the fall, my family and I went for a Sunday drive into the country, exploring antique stores. While looking for a desk for my office, I recognized the dentist's wife as she was eyeing some Lenox teacups. I barely recognized her husband. He had shrunken to half his size. He was stooped over, examining an old mortar and pestle, wearing a crumpled straw hat from an earlier century.

"Dr. S., it's good to see you," I greeted him.

When he finally looked up he had a puzzled expression on his face because he did not recognize me. His wife, who stood by, swiftly broke in and said, "You remember the doctor, dear?"

"Oh, yes, of course. I was so engrossed in this pestle. Forgive me. I once wanted to be a pharmacist, and now I collect mortars and pestles. We haven't seen you for a while Doctor."

"How are you feeling?" I finally asked. That is always a difficult question to pose to a patient whom one has not seen for a long time. After all, the dentist did have bizarre symptoms which I had attributed to drug addiction, but was that the entire story? Was there one more test to be done that I had left out? Did he see another doctor who had made a different diagnosis from mine, had found a hidden cancer or brain tumor? Sending a patient to a psychiatrist makes the assumption that there are no physical ailments accounting for the person's symptoms. It is much easier for a physician to make a positive diagnosis—neurocirculatory asthenia, muscle spasms, or the common hypoglycemia—to explain depression. It is far easier to prescribe a placebo or vitamins to "place the metabolism back in balance," rather than refer a patient to a psychiatrist. Patients resent doctors for telling them it is all in their heads. Doctors, in turn, rightfully fear that they have missed a medical explanation. Diseases such as cancer may have long incubation periods that make the patients feel sickly, and years later, when the ugly head of cancer emerges, the doctor is accused of missing a diagnosis and has to defend himself in court. It was with great trepidation that I had asked, "How are you feeling?"

"I feel the same," he said. "The psychiatrist gave me some pills for my depression, and they made me feel better for a while, and then I stopped going to him. The psychiatrist said I was worn out from thirty years of practice and it was time to quit. I don't feel like that at all. I love my work and won't quit, but I am taking it easier. I will be calling you again, Doctor. It is time for me to have a checkup."

Many months later, the dentist arrived at my office wearing a cowboy hat, knickers, and a safari shirt. He greeted me affectionately, smilingly. He was bent to one side, like the leaning tower of Pisa.

"He wants to go on a safari, and we need some shots for yellow fever, typhoid, tetanus, cholera, smallpox," his wife said. She gave me a worried glance, and I understood she wanted to talk to me alone. My nurse escorted the dentist into an examining room while I stayed behind with his wife.

"He is acting more strangely than ever. I don't know what to do with him. I'm afraid to go anywhere with him. He is on a hat kick. He buys and wears every conceivable type of hat you can imagine. This week it is the cowboy hat. Last week it was the African pith helmet. The closets are overflowing with his hats. There is no room left in the bedroom. The living room looks like a hat depository." I tried desperately to contain myself because I suddenly pictured miles and miles of hats in their apartment, stacked like a crazy cabbage field.

"When we are away from his office for a few days, he begins to act a little more normal."

"What about his leaning to one side. When did that start?" I asked.

"Only a few days ago," she said, "but every day there is something else. Yesterday he walked around with his neck twisted and his head bent over like a figure in a Mondrian painting. Last week he dragged his leg as if it were paralyzed, but when I asked him if there was anything wrong, he became angry and abusive and started accusing me of sleeping with the mailman. Doctor, my husband has become a madman. I just don't know what to do."

He was sitting on my examination table, his body angled as if he were suspended to one side of a rolling ship. His shirt was off, but he still wore his large Texan hat which was partially covering his eyes. He held a handkerchief in his hand, wiping his mouth constantly, as if he had just finished eating a succulent fruit. He sat quietly, as if in a trance, waiting to be examined. The room stank from body odor. And there was something else, some other smell I couldn't identify. His eyes were closed and he swayed back and forth—like a Buddhist monk in deep prayer.

The examination was entirely normal, except that his blood pressure was low. I placed a tongue depressor in his mouth, which was filled with saliva, and I was astounded at the decrepit condition of his teeth. His gums were red and swollen and bled at the slightest touch. His mouth looked as though he were suffering from scurvy. His tongue was coated with a white, thick cast that looked like a map—what physicians call a "geographic tongue." Did this dentist ever go to see a dentist? Doctors, after all, sometimes get the worst medical care because they diagnose themselves.

Usually, during an examination, I try to carry on some light banter to break the terrible fear the patient often feels, aware that in a minute's time something fatal could be discovered. Many patients scrutinize every crease in the doctor's face, looking for some sign that will yield a clue about what the doctor thinks. A careless sigh, a nod, or a shake of the head, can put the patient in a frenzy. What did he discover? Others, as they are unclothed, fear their innermost secrets will be discovered. But this patient was a mannequin. His skin had a sickly appearance, like lava from a volcanic terrain—wrinkled, dry, uneven, dead.

He sat clutching the table as if at any moment he were going to be torn away. I asked him to stretch out his hands as part of the neurological examination. He hesitated, but slowly released the edge of the table. His hands began to shake like leaves in the wind. (Uncontrolled tremors have many causes, well known to the physician, anywhere from rare neurological disorders to the too-familiar Parkinson's disease.)

When I finished the examination, I was as baffled as before. There were no new findings, except the disgusting state of his mouth and the conspicuous tremor. Many more tests followed, including brain scans, and he was referred to an expert neurologist who decided he was suffering from a degenerative nerve disease of unknown cause, and that there was no treatment.

His wife told me that not only was he dreadfully depressed, but he also suffered severe memory loss. Besides forgetting names of people, he had begun to have difficulty recognizing familiar things. He no longer was able to retain any new information, even forgetting who was president.

In spite of his wife's insistence that he stop, he continued to practice dentistry for a few hours a day. There was no agency or mechanism to prevent him from doing this. I wondered how he could work with those shaking hands and why patients still kept going to him. Some had been with him for twenty years or more, and they must have felt a loyalty that went beyond common sense. In those years the spectre of malpractice was rare. Patients trusted their doctors more and rarely dreamed of legal suits. Or had the lawyers simply not yet discovered that new source of wealth?

His wife was at her wit's end. Her husband refused further medical advice and insisted that he was well. What made matters worse was that he was "hopelessly absentminded," as she put it so discreetly. Because of his severe memory loss, constant arguments followed one after the other. He forgot everything his wife told him and insisted she never had. He misplaced bank statements and accused his wife of stealing from his savings accounts. He called the police, claiming he was robbed, and accused his devoted dental assistant. They found the money in his laboratory where he made his dental impressions and mixed his fillings.

"Well, you know him well enough, Doctor. You are the only one I can turn to. He trusts you. Perhaps you could go and see for yourself. Maybe there is something you can recommend. His behavior is so bizarre that I'm beginning to become a little afraid of him. It's comical and tragic to see him buy a new hat. He wears them in his office, to the amazement of the patients who think it is cute, which he claims takes the dreariness out of going to the dentist. His memory is going, but his intellect remains keen."

It was clear how desperate she was, obviously playing a charade for the rest of the world, covering up his illness. Today he probably would be diagnosed as having Alzheimer's disease, and it would not be a secret. It wouldn't have to be.

The waiting room of the dentist was large enough to seat six. Outdated magazines were strewn on a battered triangular table that held a Tiffany lamp. The walls were lined with posters declaring the importance of dental hygiene, and the nondescript dentist-office music filled the room. The chairs looked like they had been purchased from the Salvation Army of another century and were worn and decrepit—and as unsteady as the dentist.

When I arrived at the window of the cage—the cage separates patients from their destiny—there was no receptionist because she was helping the mad scientist. I coughed and knocked on the door, and out came a pleasant-looking woman.

The dentist came to the waiting room wearing a triangular hat worn by the Spanish military police on patrol. He also wore a short white coat that reached a pair of brown military pants. His high-heeled boots made him look taller.

"Welcome, good Doctor. What an honor to finally reciprocate. Now you are on my turf. When was the last time you had your teeth looked at, or cleaned?" He continued in this way as he escorted me into the inner sanctum. There were two dental chairs in two separate rooms. There was a patient in one of the rooms in a ridiculously helpless position, his mouth wide open and two suction tubes inside—a Mardi Gras mask. The office was filthy, especially the rugs, which were stained by chemical spillage. There was a disgusting odor in the office that seemed mixed with alcohol and something else, which again I didn't recognize.

"Before we begin, let me show you my office. I know my wife put you up to this, but I am glad you are here." He escorted me to his private office, which was the size of a bathroom with a small desk and two chairs surrounded by his ancient diplomas and state license to practice dentistry. Here the rug was not soiled. We moved on. "And this is the lab where I am proud to say I do all my own impressions and make my own fillings."

The lab area looked like it had never been cleaned. A long marble table was stacked with small jars and unstoppered bottles and small round crucibles for mixing the fillings. The dentist was a slob. He was in such a hurry to prepare the fillings that he bothered little with the proprieties of cleanliness. His office cleaning service was worthless. Here, that pervasive, disgusting odor suffused everything.

I suddenly realized that the solution to the medical mystery of the Mad Hatter was right here, on his workbench. The very substance from which he forged his living was now destroying his life. The culprit that was destroying his brain cells and changing this mild man into a paranoid maniac was shiny and silvery, glittering under the fluorescent light like a holy jewel. There, sitting on the counter, was the unstoppered bottle of silvery slime which, when dropped from any height, formed its own shape. And it gives off an odorless and deadly fume that slowly creeps into the body and makes its home there, a living and destroying parasite. So powerful is this chemical that when spilled on a surface, such as a rug, it can remain there for years, softly doing its treacherous work, especially in this poorly ventilated office which had become the dentist's tomb. The dentist prepared his fillings with the amalgam of silver mixed with this poisonous substance called mercury.

Mercury has been a constituent of drugs for centuries, used in antiseptics, antibacterials, diuretics, skin ointments, and laxatives. Chronic exposure to mercury in the surrounding air after inadvertent spills in poorly ventilated rooms, produces toxic effects such as the dentist was suffering. For example, the Mad Hatter in Lewis Carroll's *Alice in Wonderland* embodied the hazards of mercury used in the felt hat industry more than a hundred years ago. Major incidents of human poisoning from the inadvertent consumption of mercury-treated seed grain has occurred in Iraq, Pakistan, and Guatemala. The most notable catastrophic outbreak occurred in Iraq in 1972, resulting from the importation of large quantities of wheat and barley that had been pre-treated with mercury. Six thousand victims were hospitalized, and five hundred died.

I explained this and more to the dentist and his wife, and the following day he agreed to have his blood and urine tested for mercury.

The blood tests revealed the concentration of mercury to far exceed the normal level. We also found mercury in his hair, which was absolute proof that he was suffering from chronic mercury poisoning. The mercury vapors had concentrated in his brain, in his kidneys, and in his red blood cells.

The dentist was hospitalized and received an antidote called dimercaprol, given to him by intramuscular injections over a ten-day period. With each day, the miracle of medical treatment began to appear. His tremors decreased, his memory partially returned, his paranoid behavior subsided. I had not anticipated that such a full reversal of this very sick man's symptoms would occur, but it did.

It has reliably been reported that depression was, at one time, not uncommon among dentists, and that there were many suicides. We know now that most of these were attributable not to purely psychiatric causes but to mercury poisoning, to those little pools of silver invading human tissue.

The Mad Hatter, our dentist, is mad no longer. The noxious vapors have been dispersed. Fresh air invigorates his body and his mind, and he now gets regular dental checkups.

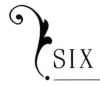

SIX

The Man with the Dark Sunglasses

By four o'clock in the afternoon there is a calm that falls into my office like a soft spring rain after a long day of listening to other people's troubles. This day was particularly tiring, and I was relieved that there was only one more patient to see.

He was a giant, muscular, man, wearing dark sunglasses, and a black striped suit, meticulously groomed and even slightly perfumed. He held his head high, towering over me regally.

After reviewing the questionnaire he had filled out, I asked him in a quiet tone, "Your name is John Rawlins?"

He nodded silently.

"Your problem is chest pain?"

"I had chest pain last night, and the emergency room doctor gave me your name. You are a heart specialist, aren't you?"

"What kind of chest pain was it?"

His answers came swift and precise, as if they were all prepared in advance. He sat perfectly straight with his hands folded on his lap.

"Why do you wear sunglasses when you are not outside in the sun?"

"The light hurts my eyes." With his huge hands, he reluctantly removed them, as an Arab woman would slip her veil down her face.

His eyes were large, round, penetrating, and as red as a glowing sunset. The lower eyelids were swollen and hanging.

It was his chest pain that he came for, not his eyes, he reminded me.

"Are you married?"

He told me he was married and had one teenage boy and one infant and worked in a warehouse, and for the past two days he had slept little because of the chest pain.

Examining this giant man was no small chore. The leads from the electrocardiograph barely reached his arms and legs, and his body extended far beyond the examining table. No hospital bed would be long enough for him.

From somewhere in the past, I remembered the fat lady who weighed 600 pounds. Four orderlies had to lift her onto two hospital beds placed side by side.

On his body were dozens of strange tattoo marks—serpents, howling wolves displaying treacherous mouths full of teeth, and skeletons. Around his bull neck hung a leather pendant with a shiny small bone.

The man kept his eyes closed and remained motionless while the nurse gently drew blood from his arm. He looked like Queequeg lying asleep.

I asked him when the tattoo marks had been burned into his skin. For the first time, he gave a broad grin and said, "In the Navy. I was on a ship that stopped in Cyprus, and a Turkish lady put them on when I was a little drunk. I was much younger then."

Back in my consulting room, I informed him that his heart was fine and asked if he had any personal troubles.

"We all have troubles, Doc," he answered. His eyes saddened, and he replaced his sunglasses.

"Do you believe," he hesitated, then asked in a soft almost childish tone, "that a man sometimes does something that he has no control over? I mean . . . there's some force that pushes things out of you and there's nothing you can do to hold it back. Nothing!"

"Yes, but why do you ask?"

"Just asking. I always liked to ask questions of people who are smarter than me—who know more. A doctor knows a lot. At school, I used to ask so many questions, it would annoy the teacher. I was born in a small southern town. My father had a farm, and there were eight of us, and we all had to work the farm. When the farm could no longer feed us, I quit school and came up here."

He had started to talk freely now that his sunglasses were on again.

"I wanted to be a doctor once, especially after I saw my mother dying of a tumor. I wanted to help."

"It's not too late, you know. You're only thirty-two. I know some people who went back to school at forty and became doctors."

"It's too late," he said in a grim, gloomy voice.

The clock struck five.

"Come back next week and let's see how your pains are doing. If they become worse, just call me."

As he rose from the chair, I was struck once more by how tall this man was. He held out a huge hand and shook my hand.

"Thank you for listening, Doc."

I made some notes in the chart and felt an uneasiness about John Rawlins. My uneasiness continued throughout the rest of the evening. At three o'clock in the morning, the insufferable phone rang. Twenty years of medical practice and I still despised that early hour call that usually summons me to the emergency room and another catastrophe in the making.

No one has yet explained why people tend to die in the early hours of the morning, especially heart patients. Perhaps that's why some of my older patients don't sleep at night, as if they know death waits for them.

"Sorry to disturb you, Doctor. This is Sergeant Bernaldo. Do you have a patient by the name of John Rawlins?"

"Yes, John Rawlins came to see me for the first time this afternoon. What happened? Is he dead?"

I could have saved his life, I thought, if I had paid more attention to his chest pain. Perhaps I should have admitted him to the hospital and spent more time examining him.

"Would you mind coming down to his house, Doc? He's not dead, if that's what you're worried about, but we need you here."

"Can't you explain what happened?"

"You'd better come down, if you don't mind."

The neighborhood was old and filled with stale odors. Police cars and two ambulances stood in front of one house, and I knew that was where John Rawlins must live. How long was it since I had made a house call?

My memory suddenly sharpened as I recalled the first time, eighteen years earlier, when I was as crisp and shiny as my alligator bag. A small man, a gnome, had called the emergency service because he couldn't breathe. It was also a hot summer night. The man was perfectly fine, just scared to be alone.

"I am the doctor," I told the officer standing on the stairs.

"Just go straight up, Doc. They're waiting for you."

The apartment door was closed with two more policemen

standing guard with long rifles. Inside the small room that served as a living room and kitchen sat John Rawlins, stiff and silent, still wearing his sunglasses and his suit. Next to him on the floor was a small boy, perhaps 13 or 14, surrounded by a pool of blood. I had never seen a murder victim until that moment.

"I think he's dead," the ambulance medic said.

I had to crouch down and sit on the floor in a pool of blood, like when I was a child playing in the water on the beach, in order to listen for any signs of life.

The unfortunate boy's head was partially bashed in, and some of his brain tissue was visible. He had a startled look on his young face and his eyes were still open. It was ridiculous going through the charade of conducting a heart examination on this obviously dead boy.

"Who did it?" I asked. If I looked one more time, I would become ill.

"His father," and the police officer pointed to John Rawlins. "He insisted on talking to you. He said you would understand. Did he act strange or say anything when you examined him today?" the detective asked, as if John Rawlins were not even in the room.

"Yes, he acted strange, but so do many people." I rose from the floor, which looked like a butcher's block.

Photographers were taking pictures of the weapon: a baseball bat.

The room was filled with too much death for me to stomach. His wife and other son weren't in sight. I wondered if they had run out when the killing began.

Could I, as a doctor, have prevented this? These thoughts must be in their minds; it was in mine.

"What do you need me here for?" I asked the detective in a pleading voice. I wanted to run out into my car, back to my comfortable bed, and wake up in the morning from this terrible nightmare.

"He wants to talk to you."

I turned to him.

"Why did you do this?"

His lips parted, but not another muscle of his face moved.

"I asked you, remember, if a man sometimes does something he does not have control over. A force that pushed out from the inside. There was a force inside of me, and you, Doc, looked like you understood what I meant."

"But this was your son," I screamed. "You butchered him!"

Two years passed and the memory of John Rawlins faded from my brain, until one afternoon I was called to the emergency room to see a patient suffering from chest pain. Being in practice for so many years, similar names of patients with similar problems appear in hospital beds. John Rawlins was the name of the patient lying in the small cubicle of the emergency room. Not for a second had I thought this was the same man, the murderer who, I thought, was serving a long jail sentence.

I saw his long body stretched out, his shirt off displaying the weird tattoo marks on his chest, and he still wore dark sunglasses. I should have refused to accept him as a patient and asked another physician to see him. Why should I care for a murderer? But my responsibility as a physician still came first, and the ethical question was swiftly settled in my mind.

"Hi, Doc. I had them call you. You're the only one I trust."

"How did you get out of jail?"

"The psychiatrist—a lot of legal wrangling. I'm working again. I see a shrink three times a week with my wife, but I still got that bad feeling in me—the bad feeling in my chest. Now I get pounding headaches. I thought I'd better go to the emergency room."

I examined his heart in silence, feeling repulsed as the image of his dead son came into my mind. His electrocardiogram was normal, but just to be on the safe side, I admitted him to the hospital. It turned out he had not had a heart attack, but before discharging him, I recalled that the last time he complained of chest pain, he had butchered his son.

"Where are you living now, John?"

"At home with my wife and son. We get along fine. My son was less than a year old when everything happened, so he doesn't know."

"How about your wife? How does she feel about it?"

"Well, she's 'come to terms,' as the psychiatrist says, but I still get that funny feeling inside of me, and now I have bad headaches which they called migraine in prison."

His psychiatrist came to visit him in the hospital and reassured the staff that John was now well adjusted. "His anger is controlled, and he is working steadily on his job and can be safely released."

On the night before his discharge from the hospital, John was sitting up in bed, bent over, holding his head between his hands with tears rolling in his eyes.

"I have awful pain, Doc," he cried. "I can't stand it anymore. The migraine medicine didn't work, and they won't give me morphine. I told them only morphine takes the pain away."

I examined him again but found no telltale signs of needle marks on his arms to suggest he was a drug addict yearning for morphine.

"I will lose control if the pain doesn't get better," he warned.

Two hours after he received his morphine injection, he suddenly lost the ability to see, his left arm became numb, his speech became slurred, and his tongue was hanging to the side. Migraine headaches sometimes do this, as will any narcotic drug. A neurologist and I examined him, and that night John had a CAT scan performed on his head that showed an enormous brain tumor.

"You need an operation, John," I told him when he was back in his room.

With his slurred speech, he said, "I told you there was some force that's pushing things out of me." He grabbed my hand in confidence and his eyes looked sadly at me.

He was operated on that night, but the tumor was too large to be removed. He never regained consciousness, and he died several weeks later.

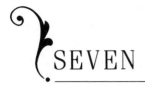

SEVEN

Fever of Unknown Origin

THE FREE STATE of Danzig was once a charming and lovely medieval city by the Baltic Sea that boasted of its magnificent old homes and brick-lined streets that dated back to the Hanseatic League.

In 1938, when I was seven years old, I lived in one of those stately homes with my parents, and a gardener, a butler, a cook, a maid, and Fräulein Marlene, my governess. The Nazification of Danzig had been completed, and the German armies would soon invade and World War II would begin.

Early in May, my parents were vacationing in Marinbaden, and I was left with Fräulein Marlene and my German shepherd, Astor. My father was a wealthy coal dealer, like his father before him. Because Jewish children were allowed to attend schools only at night, I was instructed by a tutor and rabbi who came to our home each day. Going to grade school at night was dangerous; the brown shirts prowled the streets searching for Jewish children.

My governess, Fräulein Marlene, did her best to entertain

me, but I felt crestfallen, abandoned. I began to lose my appetite, and I slept a great deal. I no longer had any desire to play in beautiful Stefan's Park with my dog.

The governess suspected that something besides loneliness and sadness was troubling me when I lost my appetite, even refusing my favorite chocolate pudding dessert at dinner one night.

"Your parents will be home soon, and it is senseless to carry on like this. You must eat something, because they will think I starved you. Tomorrow, as a treat, we will go to the docks to watch the men load the barges with your father's coal. Would you like that?"

Each day there was an exciting itinerary. I especially enjoyed visiting the famous old maritime museum, where I would see old sailing ships, and the renowned ice cream parlor, called Sprinter's, which was located on the main square. Now it was draped with huge, awesome Nazi flags, and everywhere there were brown shirts roaming around like a pack of wolves, molesting the peaceful strollers.

With Astor at my side, we walked through the winding, brick-lined streets. We finally sat at Sprinter's, which was now crowded with the terrifying white summer uniforms of the SS troops. The café had small round tables with wrought-iron chairs and colorful umbrellas. When my favorite lemon ice was brought by the waiter, I felt a wave of nauseousness. Astor gave a muffled growl whenever one of the SS men approached. They loved German shepherds, and they glanced surreptitiously at the lovely and sensuous Fräulein Marlene. She came from a long line of aristocratic Prussians and was a striking woman, with her blond hair bunched at the nape of her neck, her lustrous dark blue eyes, her head held proudly high as she ignored the Nazi ruffians who tried to get her attention.

Seeing that it was useless, that I would not even taste the

ices, we returned to our chauffeured Dusenberg parked some twenty meters from the café. We were followed by a tall uniformed German officer who approached Fräulein Marlene.

"Leaving so early, Fräulein? May I ask your name?"

Fräulein Marlene hesitated, and gave her name. "And this is my charge."

I still remember the terror of seeing the tall soldier, but Fräulein Marlene had taught me to click my heels, bow slightly, and offer an outstretched hand when greeting a stranger.

"We really must be going," she said softly. He bowed.

As soon as I climbed into the back seat, I vomited all over the brown leather; the chauffeur, Bruno, started the car in a hurry.

Every Thursday there was a Nazi rally on the main square of Danzig. Drums, flags, and thousands of people crowded to hear the speeches. On this day, the new propaganda minister, Heinrich Himmler, accompanied by Rudolf Hess, came to speak. Since the car was trapped in the crowd, we had to listen to the speeches which so appealed to most of the Danzigers— calls to unite and return to the German fatherland, to the real leader in Berlin. (Once under Prussian domain for several hundred years, Danzig, had been given to the Poles at the end of World War I. The Germans wanted it returned.)

The driver of our car pleaded to make way. "There is a sick child. Please let me pass."

Through the window, through bleary eyes, I saw children, dressed in short green pants and white shirts, waving the Nazi flags, parading and shouting, "Heil Hitler!" A giant picture of Adolf Hitler was suspended from one of the large platforms recently constructed in this beautiful and charming square, solely to conduct propaganda rallies.

On these Thursday afternoons, all the schools were closed

and the servants had their afternoons free. Fräulein Marlene would have spent the day with her friends in town were it not for my parents being in Marinbaden. Leaflets, shouting, the band playing, and the constant repetitious accusations by the frantic speakers that the Jews are enemies of the German people made me feel even sicker, and I continued to vomit until there was nothing left in my pinched stomach.

Fräulein Marlene placed her arms around me, reassured me, "Don't worry, we'll be home soon." But "soon" was three hours; it took that long to break through the tumultuous crowd which was in a fever of their own. In the car, Astor was licking my face and growling at the approach of any of the young brown shirts who threw rocks and rotten cabbage at the passing cars.

Once home, I was carried upstairs to the spacious bedroom that was enclosed by sliding doors. Astor sat and watched as Fräulein Marlene placed a thermometer underneath my armpit. My body felt on fire as my temperature registered 104. She quickly and ably covered my body with towels soaked in cool alcohol. The family doctor, Dr. Citroen, a close friend of my parents, and a renowned practitioner and professor, could not be reached. Neither could my parents.

When my temperature returned to normal in a few hours, I scrambled out of the bed and spent what was left of the afternoon in our library. It was a spacious room bedecked with Flemish tapestries; hundreds of leather-covered books lined the walls. Some of the shelves were enclosed by glass. I knew that these contained first editions of great and forbidden books. Some of the university professors would visit on Saturday afternoons, devouring the great works in the original editions— Goethe, Schiller, Heine, Schnitzler, Zweig, Verlaine, Baudelaire. This was my favorite room in the house, and I relished sitting in my father's leather chair, studying the wonderful colored pictures in *Fables of Fontaine*. The chair was part of a semi-circle, surrounding a large oak-panelled fireplace that had our family crest engraved on it.

As I stared at the book, the pages became blurred and I felt warm and started to sweat. Fräulein Marlene came storming into the library, angry that I had dared leave the bed. She brusquely carried me off into the bedroom, where I now developed a fierce headache and started to vomit greenish material. At ten o'clock in the evening Dr. Citroen arrived, wearing his usual dark blue suit, white shirt, and blue tie, and holding his doctor's bag. I saw his blurred mustached face from my bed as he opened the sliding doors, but as he was about to enter the room, Astor growled, baring his teeth. Fräulein Marlene tried to coax the dog away with meat and cookies, but to no avail. The faithful and possessive dog sat next to my bedside, utterly defiant, not allowing the doctor to come near. Astor must have sensed that I was afraid of Dr. Citroen because he had once hurt me with an injection.

My temperature began to rise, and my head felt like it was being smashed by a sledgehammer. Dr. Citroen, from the entrance of the bedroom, was calmly giving instructions to Fräulein Marlene. Each time Dr. Citroen edged his body through the rolling door, Astor charged furiously forward with every intention of biting the doctor, who then swiftly pulled the rolling door shut. He pleaded with me to somehow pacify the dog so that he could perform an examination.

Aspirin, hot tea with lemon, alcohol sponges, and tinctures of belladonna with phenobarbitol were gingerly administered to me by the governess, under the watchful eyes of Astor and Dr. Citroen.

Soon asleep—or was I hallucinating?—the room was spinning like a top, and young boys dressed in brown pants and brown shirts, wearing the Nazi armband surrounded me, shouting "Heil Hitler!" and singing the Nazi war song, the "Horst Wessel." As they goosestepped around the bed, I felt them pulling me to the floor. The Nazi emblem was placed tightly around my right arm causing the arm to ache, and then I was marching in the long playroom which was the miniature highway I used to drive the toy Dusenberg. At first I enjoyed the attention, and even joined in singing the last chorus of the "Horst Wessel," but I could not raise my legs, while the other boys kicked their legs high in the air, much as in a chorus line. Then I was on a train that arrived in America, and I was walking on the street wearing the Nazi armband as crowds of people fell away from me as I tiptoed on giant gold coins lining the streets. I became frightened and cried. A smiling bearded face appeared, placing his arms around my shoulders as Astor jumped and licked his face. The early morning light shone on Rabbi Kroll, my teacher, who was sitting on my bed.

"You had a bad dream," he gently told me. "That happens when the temperature goes too high."

Curiously, Astor allowed the rabbi into the room, but again guarded me from the doctor who arrived later in the morning. My temperature had returned to normal, I felt much stronger and I yearned for a soft-boiled egg, which Fräulein Marlene served with apple compote on a bowl of rice, and a cup of tea, and a slice of pound cake.

Dr. Citroen continued giving instructions from the partially opened door, insisting that I remain at bedrest, which I protested bitterly. I threatened to pull out all the down feathers from the pillows and bedcover and to never eat again.

By late afternoon, I felt so restless and rejected that I unbuttoned the pillowcase and pulled out the feathers one by one, flinging them into the air, then watching them float down like giant snowflakes. In no time at all, the bedroom looked like a chicken coop, feathers covered the parquet floor, the dressers, easy chairs, and Astor shaking his strong body furiously to get free of the whiteness.

My Uncle Hermann came to visit and roared hysterically as he saw the bedroom, a blanket of feathers. Astor greeted him with wagging tail and jumped on him to lick his face.

"He's not sick, for heaven's sake. He misses his parents, that's all. Let him out of bed."

Uncle Hermann was a jovial man, round as a gourd, with a gregarious pumpkin smile. He was unmarried and lived with a German woman. His business was money exchange. He was the renegade of the family, refusing to enter the family's coal and wood enterprises. On Saturday afternoons he used to take me to the art cinema to see the Katzenheimmer Kids cartoons, then we'd stop at Rosenbaum's department store for toys, and then we'd end the afternoon at Sprinter's ice cream parlor. Not only was he my uncle, he was also my best friend. (He refused to leave Danzig with us when we made our escape from Gestapo headquarters. In 1945, at the end of the war, the Allies found him hanging from the entrance gate of Dachau, over a sign that read, "Work Makes Free." The story goes that he had escaped from three concentration camps and was finally caught smuggling food into Dachau the day before the liberation and quickly and brutally hanged.)

As was his custom, he brought a present for me, and from his baggy pocket there emerged a small crystal radio and a tiny sailing ship, a replica of one of the Hanseatic League ships of the 1400s. But with all his coaxing and pleading with me, he could not get Astor to leave the room.

By nightfall, my temperature again rose, this time to 105 degrees, and I was again taking my hallucinatory trips. This time, I was on the main street of Danzig, and the brown-shirt boys were running after me, shouting, "Kill the Jew!" and reciting Himmler's monstrous litany, "The Jews are our misfortunes. They starve us. They killed Jesus Christ."

Between my bouts of hallucinations, I heard Dr. Citroen say to the governess, "We'll have to put the dog away, because otherwise the boy will die."

"That we cannot do," she answered.

"Fräulein, we have no choice. His parents won't be here until the morning. That may be too late. He is probably suffering from meningitis. We have to put him into the hospital."

In my crepuscular condition, I leaned down towards the floor and found Astor's collar, pulled him into the bed, and firmly placed my arms around his thick neck.

In the early hours of the morning, Fräulein Marlene was sitting in an armchair adjacent to the bed, wearing a nightgown and robe, in a deep sleep. All of my bones felt stiff and painful, as if somebody had put them in a vise. I crawled out of bed, moving my body like a caterpillar, heading towards the bathroom. A flickering morning light shone into the room as I watched the rolling doors slowly open. The gardener, standing watch by the door, rushed into the room and reached for Astor. Astor attacked him, and he shrieked so loudly that the governess leapt from the chair, while I kept crawling to the bathroom to vomit.

Several men were now standing by the rolling doors carrying a large net. Astor crawled on the floor next to me. "That will never work," Fräulein Marlene shouted as I reached the toilet bowl.

By late morning, my parents returned from Marinbaden. They brought me a large toy bear wearing a red cap. He was as tall as I, and Astor liked licking his paws. My mother, who looked tanned and rested, started to cry when she saw my pale, drawn face.

"I had a feeling we should have come back sooner," she

yelled at my father. "He is half the size he was when we left."

After my father removed Astor from the bedroom, Dr. Citroen examined me thoroughly but he could not find the cause of the fever. "Perhaps the beginning of measles or mumps, and after the fever drops, the rash may appear," he told them. "Don't worry, young lad. Soon you will be running at your old tricks."

For the next two days, I felt fine and was allowed out of bed. I stayed in my playroom most of the day, furiously driving the toy Dusenberg from end to end. The big bear, whom I called Meyer, after our milkman who was very hairy and dark looking, sat in the back of the car. He was an exact replica of the dancing bear who entertained in the nightclubs in Berlin. (The dancing bears were the rage of Germany in the Thirties, as was sniffing cocaine. So too, was Berthold Brecht, who was appreciated selectively—who heeded his "message"?)

At the end of my playroom were large French doors that opened to a magnificent stone balcony that had two lion heads at each end. The balcony looked upon Stefan's Park which had beautiful circles of hundreds of tulips forming the design of the Danzig emblem—two eagles on each side of a shield. By the end of spring, they were replaced by hundreds of poppies, foxglove, geraniums, and begonias. Beyond the flower beds, there was a soccer field. But there was no soccer being played anymore.

By the fourth day, my temperature reappeared in the same furious fashion, preceded by shaking chills and a great deal of fatigue, and again I slipped into a semi-stupor.

Dr. Citroen sat by the bedside, soaking my body with alcohol and administering various drugs that only made me drowsier. At the end of the week, there was still no rash and the fever continued. My body was saturated with aspirin to relieve joint pains. Perhaps rheumatic fever was the cause of all these fevers; Dr. Citroen did hear a slight heart murmur, but it was not the cause of my distress.

Between the bouts of fever and semi-starvation, I felt extraordinarily weak. Mother sat by me night and day, and father came home each night with another new surprise.

One day after the fourth week, sitting in the playroom, I heard drums and marching through the window. There were hundreds of boys in brown uniforms, carrying large posters, praising the glory of Adolf Hitler and viciously cursing the Jews. There were terrible, sickening pictures depicting Jews draining the blood from German babies.

They marched and crushed the tulips and geraniums, leaving behind a flattened field of dirt. As helpless onlookers observed with great despair, it was as if an army of locusts had infested the fields. Some parents ran out towards their marching children, trying to retrieve them, but the tall brown-shirt leaders held them back.

"You should be proud of your sons," they yelled. "Don't try to disrupt the march. These are the young children who belong to the Führer. They are no longer yours."

We all stood on the balcony—my mother and father, Fräulein and the butler—watching this madness develop and strengthen, none of which I could really understand.

"Why do they hate us so much?" I asked my father, who answered by placing his arms snugly around me.

Through the doors, I heard my mother and father arguing that it was no longer safe to stay in Danzig, and that we should leave for Switzerland.

"It will blow over, as every pogrom. How can we leave everything?" he said.

"Then I'll go to Switzerland with our son."

My physical condition was deteriorating, and Uncle Hermann insisted I be taken to see the famous Dr. Sauerbruch a visiting professor, from Maine at the Wilhelm Hospital in Berlin. "If you don't take him, I'll take him myself." He made the arrangements in his usual clever way.

Dr. Citroen feared I might be suffering from childhood leukemia because the white blood-cell count was high, but there were no other signs of the illness.

The following morning we were at the majestic-looking Victorian railroad station, built in 1890 under the Prussian empire. There were special Fiat carriages bedecked in red that were reserved for the nobility of Europe who came to the seaside resort of Sopot to gamble at the casino or to stroll on the famous boardwalk, the longest in Europe. Now these special carriages carried the SS troops and diplomats. The train station was crowded with German soldiers and hundreds of Jews who were escaping to Warsaw.

My father arranged for us to travel in one of those splendid carriages, which contained a bedroom and living room, and we had our own private waiter. The walls were upholstered with blue and red velvet; there were large comfortable chairs resting on Persian rugs. The morning train to Berlin was bustling with activity. My mother saw some of her friends—lawyers, judges, professors—who were escaping from Danzig to go to Warsaw.

"We should be going with them," she told my father.

Fräulein Marlene was with us, and my father whispered, "There is no escaping. If the war comes, Warsaw will be one of the worst places."

He had made arrangements to leave for Switzerland if the political situation worsened. (Switzerland allowed just a trickle of Jews to enter their country, but my father also had alternative plans in case the Swiss backed down.)

I sat on one of the lush chairs by the window as the train snaked along the sea edge, and I saw the white silky beach, the famous Seestern Café, and the Casino Park with all the yew trees and donkey carts. How I wished that I had the strength to run on the beach and ride the donkey!

The Berlin train, a German train, made a stop in Warsaw, letting off the Jews with all their belongings that they could carry themselves. Polish soldiers came on the train, making a scrupulous examination of everybody's passports, looking with scorn at the SS. For the time being, they were still in control.

Our next-door neighbor, Prince B. of Danzig, came into our carriage and played bridge with my parents. He was one of the many Germans who hated the Nazis and befriended Jews. (He was a homosexual—almost as bad as being a Jew— and, within two years, he would be found hanging in his bathroom closet.)

"What hotel will you be staying at?" he asked my mother.

"The only place we could get in is the Schweitzerhoff."

The prince had a peculiar look on his face. "You mean the Schweitzerhoff at Wilhelm Plaza?"

"Yes. What's wrong with the hotel?"

The prince said no more. They sat by the card table and played bridge for the rest of the night and drank champagne.

I slept through most of the trip. We arrived in Berlin in the late evening. The hotel was a ten-minute walk from the hospital. An appointment was made with Dr. Sauerbruch at nine o'clock sharp in the morning, in his office. One of my father's business associates picked us up and drove us in his Mercedes to the Schweitzerhoff Hotel. Drowsy and feeling weak, my father wanted to carry me, but I stubbornly insisted on walking into the hotel.

Inside, there were hundreds of people in formal dress, and the SS dressed in black uniforms. By every door, as if they were stuck to the wall, were German soldiers carrying rifles with bared bayonets. I looked up towards the ceiling which was covered with gold angels, birds and painted gardens.

"It looks like we walked into a big party," Fräulein Marlene said, holding onto my hand.

The crowd was so thick that we could not approach the registration desk. Suddenly, the crowd parted and formed a path on either side, as crowds of men with German shepherds marched into the hotel. They surrounded a man who was smiling, wearing baggy pants and a raincoat. He was flanked by Rudolf Hess, and by the squirrel-looking man who was the propaganda minister, Joseph Goebbels.

The crowd went into a frenzy, shouting "Seig Heil!" as the mustached man slowly walked down the line of people with a warm smile and outstretched arm.

Fräulein Marlene, my father, my mother and I stood frozen. The man with the mustache and the raincoat stopped short in front of us.

"So late," he laughed and rubbed his hands together, and then stroked my hair. "A good German lad should be at home in bed."

I recognized the man with the mustache from the posters. I felt my face brighten red, and my heart raced like a train. Lightbulbs flashed, and then there was applause as he and his entourage disappeared into the elevator. Curious reporters came running up, asking, "What did he say to you?"

After this brief encounter, the concierge, Hans Schneider, personally escorted us to our rooms upstairs. Throughout the night my body was shaking and trembling from the temperature and the strange feelings I experienced, seeing the leader of Germany. The Danzig newspaper the following morning reported the incident with a picture of us and Hitler on the front page.

At eight o'clock in the morning, a taxicab drove us to the Wilhelm Hospital where I was escorted to a private room. My parents were asked to leave, as was Fräulein Marlene. Never had I felt so abandoned and frightened; I began immediately to plan my escape. I searched the walls, which were painted white, and on one side, in a brown frame, hung the picture of Adolf Hitler.

A nightstand was adjacent to the bed, with a large silver tray covered by a white napkin. There were four gruesome-looking syringes with long needles, test tubes snugly placed side by side, along with a jar of round white cottonballs immersed in alcohol. The bed stood high off the ground and was covered with a thin white blanket with a black Nazi emblem in its center. The door was locked, and I pushed one of the wooden chairs next to the window which was partially open. Outside, there was a narrow circular ledge which was large enough to stand on. It was covered with thick ivy that fell to the ground, where there was a narrow walk lined with pebbles. A large lawn was in front. Patients were sitting in wheelchairs and benches.

I crouched down and edged my body underneath the window, but suddenly I felt a pair of thick hands pull me around my waist and swing me in the air.

"What are you doing here, for heaven's sake?" a loud coarse voice came from the nun who was going to be my nurse. She was the biggest woman I had ever seen, wearing a large white triangular hat with a black cross between two large breasts.

"Get undressed immediately!" she screamed. She closed the window and locked it, and her eyes glared at me furiously.

"For a sick child," she yelled, "you behave like one of those ruffians."

Quickly, I undressed down to my shorts. I was too frightened to do otherwise, and I was too embarrassed to go further. She threw me a white hospital gown. "Put this around you before you get even sicker."

She picked me up and placed me down on the bed. As I scrambled out of my underpants, I felt a greasy thermometer enter into my backside.

"Don't move," she said, "or we'll chain you to the bed."

I lay still as a rock, as images of chains appeared in front of my face, my arms and legs attached to the bedpost. Squeezing my hand tightly on the edge of the bed, even at the risk of death, I refused to allow myself to cry. Those large hands rolled me on my back, and she kept repeating, "Make one move and you will be a sorry one, you will be."

Minutes later, a cheerful blond-haired doctor came into the room, as happy as if he had come to a birthday party. "Well now, our Danzig kid, we are going to take some blood from your arm, and tomorrow morning Dr. Sauerbruch will come and talk to you and examine you."

The doctor's face above me looked like white marble with blue eyes and blond hair glued onto his head. "Close your eyes and you'll feel just a tiny stick, and if you move I know I will hurt you." At that point I resigned myself to become a statue for the rest of my stay in the hospital.

He placed a tourniquet around my arm which pinched my skin and continued asking me questions about *schlagball*, handball, and soccer which every schoolchild played. Soccer was my forté. Being small and quick, I could race around the field and easily dodge the taller boys. I watched the long needle slowly enter into my vein, making that certain sound I will always remember. He pulled back on the lever and the syringe filled with blood. The whole process so fascinated me—the blood leaving the arm and then seeping up into the syringe—that I forgot to cry. He continued smiling with his perfect mannequin face. I wondered at that time if he would be smiling if I did the same to him.

"We are going to see if your blood is filled with little bugs, which may be in your body and make you sick."

As he said that, I pictured thousands of bugs swarming through my body, climbing into my nose, ears, head, and mouth, and the thought nauseated me. I remembered seeing bugs once at a refugee camp in Danzig, a camp sponsored by Jewish organizations throughout the world to help poor Jews leave Europe and go to America. My mother, a volunteer, took me one morning to see what it was like in these embarkment camps. In one of the barracks where the people slept on wooden cots, I saw bugs crawling over the floors and on the beds and the dinner trays. I wondered if these were the same bugs swarming in my body.

The narrow brown tourniquet around my arm began to prick but I was afraid to tell him that I was in so much pain. He was so busy transferring the blood from the syringe into the test tube before the blood clotted that he forgot to remove the tourniquet. My arm began to turn blue, and I finally cried out in pain.

"It's all right, Danzig kid. You're a good boy. You don't have to cry. We have other Jewish boys here, you know, but they aren't as brave as you."

He saw that the tears were rolling down my face which was twisted like an accordion, and I pointed to my right arm. He swiftly released the tourniquet and my arm turned a bright red. The nun stood by with an expression of some pleasure in her eyes, especially since I finally let myself go and cried without stopping.

"Can I see my mother?" I begged the nun. "I want to go home."

"Don't try it," she said. "The windows in the room are locked, and I will be checking you every hour." She placed a long hard index finger at the crease of my elbow which was covered with a piece of cotton.

"Now give me a sample of urine," she demanded, again in a harsh voice.

"I can't go now."

"You'd better, or I'll force a tube into your pee-pee."

Now I was certain I had to plan an escape from this horrid woman.

"Come into the bathroom, you little Jew devil," she yelled. "Take this bottle and concentrate."

She turned the faucet on in the sink as my body began to shake. The night temperature was on the rise and I developed a shaking chill. The blond doctor returned.

"We'd better do a spinal tap on him. He may be suffering from meningitis. Please bring me the spinal tray, nurse," he said to the nun.

Whatever it meant, it sounded horrible, and I began to scream. Long needles and sheets of linen were brought into the room by an orderly who proceeded to tie my hands and legs like a mummy. My back was arched like a boomerang as the orderly and the nun grasped me in a wrestling hold. I felt a cold solution soak my back.

"Hand me the syringe," the doctor said. It was one of those long ugly-looking needles that was going to be placed into my spine.

As the nun handed the instrument to the doctor, he kept calling me the brave Danzig kid. The nun quickly said, "You know, doctor, you'd better check with Professor Sauerbruch and see if this is all right to do."

"Nurse, this is an emergency."

"I still think you ought to check with the professor. This boy was personally greeted by the Führer at the Schweitzerhoff Hotel!"

Magic! The bed ties were undone, the needle and syringe were placed back on the tray, and I became eternally grateful to the nun. Professor Sauerbruch was notified and decided not to perform the spinal tap until after he had examined me. I was given a brownish liquid solution to drink, a bromide, and minutes later I was fast asleep.

In the morning, I thought I was in my own bed in Danzig until a young nurse came into the room carrying a tray with applesauce and rice and some warm tea. My hospital gown was changed, and she was cheerful and bright.

"My name is Herta," she said, "and Professor Sauerbruch will be here in a few minutes."

I had no desire to eat but was afraid not to. The night before remained a living nightmare. Had I really seen Hitler? Had I really been tied up? I was looking for the nun who saved me from the needle stick in my spine to come into the room, and I wondered when my parents would arrive.

Herta straightened the bed covers and placed a clean towel on the night table, along with a metal tongue depressor, a flashlight, and a round headlight and earscopes.

The door of the room briskly opened and three doctors and two nurses entered, chattering. The tallest of the men was Professor Sauerbruch. He had a lean body with a narrow face and gray hair.

"I'm Dr. Sauerbruch," he gently said. As he sat down on my bed, he took one of my sweaty hands into his. "You've had a bad time, but don't worry. Soon, we'll make you better and you will be able to go back to your beautiful city, Danzig. You would like that, wouldn't you?"

I nodded.

"Do you have a dog?"

"Yes."

"And his name?"

"Astor."

"I bet he misses you. Does he sleep with you?"

"No, but he stays in the room. He's a German shepherd."

"Ah! I too, have one. His name is Bruno." I thought of our chauffeur who resembled a German shepherd. He then proceeded to ask me dozens of questions—when had I become ill, how had I felt between the times when the temperature was down, what joints hurt me, about my headaches.

"And what do you like to eat the most?"

"Chocolate pudding, soft-boiled eggs, and sauerbraten."

"How about other meat?"

"I only like *Klobsens.*"

"Do you drink milk?"

"I hate milk, especially if it's warm and has a skin on top."

"What about cheese?"

"I love cheese. I like to eat a lot of that."

"What is your favorite cheese?"

"Goat cheese. I'm the only one in the house who eats it. My Fräulein serves me goat cheese at every lunch."

"Goat cheese, then. I like it, too," he said. "Well, I'm going to now examine you." Now, looking back, I so admire his gentle bedside manner and his marvelous ability to instill confidence and make me feel secure. The great clinician of another time.

His long fingers started examining my neck, and then he placed them in my armpit looking for swollen glands, which tickled and made me giggle. He pounded on my chest and then moved his hands to my belly as he looked for the liver and spleen, which again caused convulsive laughter, which also made him laugh.

"I know I'm tickling you, but just try to think of something else so I can better feel all your organs inside that little belly."

He took a hammer from his coat pocket and tapped my knees, which responded with a quick thrust. "You're a lively one," he said.

With each minute, I became more relaxed, and I didn't mind being examined.

From his long white coat's side pocket, he produced a small piece of wood in the shape of a cylinder with a finely carved

caduceus. One end of the cylinder he placed over my heart and
bent his ear to the other. The room now was perfectly silent
as he used his ancient stethoscope, moving to the various parts
of my heart. When he was finished, he looked up and spoke.
"Do you like this instrument?"

He handed it to me, and I touched it with my hands and
placed it to my own ear.

"Now, sit up, young man. I'm going to listen to your lungs."

This time he did not use the wooden stethoscope, but placed
his naked ear against the left and right sides of my back while
he asked me to cough, and then to talk loudly, and then to
whisper. His fingers tapped up and down my chest, and when
he was finished he said, "You are going to be just fine, but we'll
have to do some more tests."

Seeing the grimace on my face, he quickly added, "But no
more needles."

After they left, from outside the half-open door, I heard
Professor Sauerbruch chatting with the other doctors, using
such words as "blood disease," "leukemia," "tuberculosis," and
"rheumatic fever."

The pretty young nurse placed me in a large wooden wheel-
chair, and wheeled me through the long white marble hospital
corridors that led to a freight elevator.

"We're going for a little ride," she said to me. "First upstairs, and then through a long tunnel into the X-ray room."

When we arrived, the room was dark and I saw Professor
Sauerbruch wearing a long lead apron, standing behind a sandy
screen.

"Now take everything off," he said, "and stand in front of
the screen. I am going to move this screen up and down so I
can see the insides of you."

"What will you see?" I asked him.

"This is a fluoroscope, and I will watch your lungs move and
your heart beat."

He scanned me for more than one-half hour, describing his findings to his nurse, who wrote them down on a clipboard. For a moment, in his large metal apron, he looked to me like a butcher in our meat store. After he had finished, he gave me a warm smile, shook my hand, and said my lungs were perfect, and soon I could climb any mountain or enter a foot race. Immediately, I pictured myself with a knapsack, racing up the Matterhorn.

After being wheeled into another room, I had to swallow a disgusting thick white liquid that made me vomit. After several words of encouragement, I tried again, because he said, "It is important that your stomach is X-rayed."

After the third attempt, I swallowed the chalky thick syrup, and the fluoroscopic examination continued. I felt the cold screen against my body. By the late morning, I returned to my hospital room and welcomed the sight of the nun. She still had a harsh look on her face, but spoke in a more gentle tone.

"You can take a nap, and then I'll bring you some lunch, and later on, another doctor is going to examine your heart." She washed me with a wet cloth and gave me a new fresh gown, and waited patiently by the bed.

Sharply at two o'clock in the afternoon, a new entourage of doctors marched into the room, headed by the chief of cardiology, Dr. Forssmann. He had jet black hair and a face like a bulldog. He looked like one of the stormtroopers who hung around the beer halls in Munich, and his manners were no different.

Without even introducing himself, in an abrupt manner, he pulled the sheets off me and placed a stethoscope on my chest, twisting his face so that he looked like the reflection in a circus mirror. (Professor Werner Forssmann was a Nazi, but will be best remembered for the remarkable feat of performing the first cardiac catheterization on himself. Under the fluoroscope, he passed a long tube into his own arm, guiding it into his heart as he watched it on the fluoroscope. A nurse and a student were at his side. He accomplished this daring feat in 1929, which really gave birth to modern cardiology and to cardiac catheterization, and which won him the Nobel Prize in 1956.)

While he listened to the heart, he closed his eyes and moved his head, as if he were listening to a concerto. When the examination was completed, he pulled the sheets back on my naked chest, rumpled my hair, and winked.

"He has a small heart murmur," he told his colleagues in the room who were waiting for the professor's diagnosis, "but it is not significant. Perhaps his parents will allow me to pass a tube into his heart."

The other men laughed at that suggestion while I was repelled with fear. Not long after that, Dr. Forssmann was dismissed from the hospital by Dr. Sauerbruch because of his experimentation on himself and his desire to perform on others as soon as possible.

In the days to follow, my parents and Fräulein Marlene came to visit as my temperature began to return to normal. On the fourth day of my hospital stay, my clothes were brought into my room, my parents dressed me, and we had a meeting in Professor Sauerbruch's office.

It was a large office with two couches and an antique desk. On the wall were dozens of pictures of doctors and prominent persons who had visited his clinic. He rose from his desk and proffered a warm handshake.

"You can take your boy home today. All our tests show that he is not suffering from leukemia, tuberculosis, or rheumatic fever. He is suffering from a rather common disease, usually not diagnosed, called brucellosis. It's a strange disease which you get from eating goat cheese. It is caused by a bacteria called the *brucella ovis*, and was discovered by a Frenchman, of course. It usually gets better by itself, but may go on for months with fever, fatigue, weight loss, and joint pains, just as it has in your son. I suspect that in another six weeks he will be completely recovered."

I will never forget the joy and happiness that shone on my parents' faces. With tears, laughter, handshakes, and lots of hugging and kissing, we were about to depart from the office when Professor Sauerbruch said, "Oh, by the way, young man, since you were so interested in this wooden stethoscope, I am going to present you with one."

He opened his drawer and pulled out a replica of the one that he was carrying. "Maybe someday you, too, will become a doctor."

To this day, I am in possession of this wooden stethoscope. It was one of the rare things that I was able to take with me when we escaped from Gestapo headquarters in 1939.

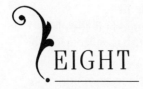

EIGHT

Leysin

THE TRAIN RIDE from Lausanne, Switzerland, to Leysin took forty-five minutes, winding through the beautiful valleys of the Swiss Alps. It was the winter of 1952, and I was on this train heading for the famous TB sanatorium. The sanatorium was located on top of one of the magnificent Alpine Mountains, and the train stopped at its base. The air here was clear and dry, and the mountain was covered by miles of sparkling white snow. Everything, including the sanatorium, was white, except for the elevator—a freight elevator that carried the dead back down the mountain to the train that would take them back to Lausanne. It looked like the freight elevator in New York that lifted cars to their parking spots.

Fifteen medical students were crowded into this vertical moving bus, which had a medicinal smell. Fifteen medical students ascended to meet TB patients for the first time. We had come to learn about the most dreadful disease of the century.

We took little notice of the beauty that surrounded us because of our fears and anxiety of what lay before us.

Not far from this sanatorium was a renowned health and ski spa where healthy people went to enjoy the pleasures of the grand tranquility of the mountains and the air.

A pleasant-looking nurse met us as we stepped off the elevator and escorted us to the lecture hall. It looked like the rotunda in most other medical schools, except this one was surrounded by glass that gave view to a white paradise of glistening snow and the awesome surrounding mountains. The lecturer who was going to give us the preliminary talk on TB was as tall as a giraffe wearing a long white coat.

"I'm Professor Michaud. I have TB, mostly cured, and I have been in this sanatorium since I was a medical student like you."

His opening remarks left us unnerved because, each year, one or more students contracted TB and was forced into a sanatorium for cure. Antibiotics for the treatment of tuberculosis had not yet been discovered. The only treatment consisted of the "open-air method." Rest and exposure to the sun, along with drastic surgical treatment, such as pumping air into the stomach or chest to collapse the diseased lung. Sometimes, attempts were made to cut the TB cavity free from the lung.

I was assigned two female patients, one was in her late sixties, and the other, Gabrielle, was twenty-three years old.

Outside on a large open terrace, patients in underclothes were strewn on long folding chairs lying in the sun like skiers resting between slaloms.

A long white corridor was lined by private patients' rooms. Each door had a plaque with the name of its tenant.

My older patient was Madame Corot, whose name was written on a small gold plaque. A pleasant voice answered after I knocked. Sitting by the window was a gray-haired woman, knitting, wearing a colorful shawl around her narrow shoulders. *"Entré.* Please come in and close the door. We don't want a draft, do we?" she said.

"I am the new medical student assigned to examine you."

"Oh, I know, it is the beginning of the month."

"You speak English very well," I told her.

"Thank you, that is a compliment coming from an American. Actually, I taught myself. I have the time to do it. Please sit down. Would you like a glass of champagne? It is nearly lunch."

"Thank you, but it is too early for me."

"Ah, yes, you Americans live by the clock. There is a time to eat, to drink, to sleep, to work, and perhaps there is a time set to die, but you are too young to understand all that." She pushed herself off the chair and walked over to the far side of the room to the shelf of a large French armoire that was stacked with champagne bottles.

As she was pouring a glass for herself my eyes roamed around the room. It was richly furnished with a dark oak table, an upholstered chair, bookshelves, a small, round, inlaid French table and a small, four-poster canopy bed covered with a red woven blanket brocaded with golden fibers. Everywhere the room was festooned with rich colors. Ottoman brocaded fabrics and silks upholstered the chairs and benches and there were spreads on the floor. On the walls hung calligraphies of embroidered silk designs displayed in vivid colors. I felt I was standing in the room of the the Sultan Sulayman from the sixteenth century.

"My family are Turks, Ottomans," she said. "I was born in Istanbul."

Outside of the room was a large balcony with a blue velvet chaise loungue covered by a large canvas to protect it from the rain.

"We have to sit outside on the balcony three hours a day, and when the weather permits, the doctor asks us to sleep outside several times a week, but I am getting too old for these outside acrobatics.

"Now, my young American student, take a chair here and I will answer your questions while I drink my champagne."

With pad and pencil in hand I started the routine of taking a medical history.

"How old are you?"

"The last time I counted I was 61. If it weren't for you students, I would have lost count long ago."

"When was the first time you became ill?"

"Thirty-five years ago, before you were born."

"You have had TB for thirty-five years?"

"Perhaps longer. I was married and lived in the Topkapi Palace in Istanbul. When my child was six years old I became ill."

"How long have you been in Leysin?"

"Twenty-five years. The doctors said I was not to leave if I wanted to stay alive." She continued to talk without my asking her questions, and after one hour, and ten pages of scribbled notes, she said, "I am getting tired. Let us continue tomorrow. It is time for lunch. They will serve it in my chambers, and then I will have a nap, and it will be time for you to take the train back to Lausanne."

The students ate lunch in a common cafeteria used for the staff and visitors. Actually, it was a full dinner that included wine, soup, pork chops, mashed potatoes and a Napoleon dessert and coffee. Each of the students sitting at my table were relating their first encounters with their TB patients. At first I was reluctant to eat any of the food because the TB bacilli pervaded everywhere in this beautiful setting. But as no one else seemed to share my fears, I ate a delicious meal all for one dollar and thirty cents.

After lunch I went to visit the next patient. Her room was located on the other side of the hospital, at the end of a long hall that smelled of oxalic acid disinfectant. This was the home of the very sick patients, some who were waiting to die.

One of the students informed me that the disinfectant had seeped into the hall from one of the rooms where a patient had died. It had been cleaned and made ready for the next tenant. A stretcher passed covered with a white sheet, carrying one of the dead. They were carried down to the basement where an autopsy was performed. Then they were placed in a sealed brown box and taken down the mountain in the elevator to a special compartment train and back to their homes to be buried. The coffin was not opened again because the TB was still alive in the dead patient.

Here, the patients had numbers, not names, on their doors. After knocking on the door there was no response, and I meekly opened it. Inside there was a bed with a young woman lying in it covered with a white sheet. Her eyes were closed, and she had long beautiful brown hair spread out on a large pillow like a fan. As I was about to leave she spoke in a sweet French voice, "Don't go away. I was only resting. I become so tired after lunch. I was outside all day on the deck. I hate being inside when the sun is out. Are you one of the doctors?"

My ability to speak French was improving, but I still carried a very strong accent. "I am one of the students, here to examine you."

The room was stark and depressing. There was nothing in the room except a bed, a night table and a commode with an empty urinal on the floor. A clipboard hung from the wall, keeping a daily record of the patient's temperature. With my other patient, I had felt intimidated by the luxurious surrounding. Madame Corot had been well indoctrinated by the hundreds of medical students who had visited her, but this poor young soul was afraid, shy, and vulnerable. She lay helpless in the bed like a wounded bird, and she appeared so desperately pale I was afraid she was going to die in front of me, something I could not bear to witness. Gently, ever so softly, I moved the bare chair next to her bed. "I am an American medical student. My French is very bad so be patient with me, and don't speak too fast, because then I won't understand you and you will have to repeat everything again."

She laughed. "I can understand you. Don't be afraid of me. You can sit down. I won't make you sick, but if I become tired you will have to come back tomorrow."

She must have seen the apprehension on my face and the pity in my eyes. Finally, I sat on the chair, sniffing the air, which smelled of the disinfectant rising from the floor.

"They just scoured the floor with that disgusting fluid," Gabrielle said. "It is good to rest. I was outside all morning where the air was fresh, so fresh that it made my body tired. I must be very sick," she sadly said. "Everyday I look to be stronger; instead I feel worse. Is that what is supposed to happen?"

"It takes time to get better. You must be patient," I told her in an unconvincing voice.

"How old are you?" I started on the traditional routine of history taking.

"Twenty-three." Her eyes were like two light amethysts, soft, transparent like the faint lines of a Dégas painting.

"How long have you been ill?"

"I am not sure. It was so long ago." Her cheeks were pale except for two jolly red circles. She kept tugging at the sheets to bring them up to her narrow neck, as if to hide the rest of her.

"I became ill on Easter day with a bad cold and it didn't improve. My father took me to the doctor and they X-rayed my chest and here I am. Simple as that. So it must be six months. Time stands still on the mountains; only the light changes." As she spoke her voice was interrupted by a violent cough and then she began to wheeze.

"Are you all right?" I asked.

"I start to cough when I speak too long. I used to love to talk, sometimes too much. When I lived at home with my parents and two younger sisters, they complained that I never stopped chatting. 'You are a chatterbox,' my mother told me."

"Are you a student?" I asked.

"Yes, I dance."

Her face became violaceous red, the color of begonias in bloom. "It must be early afternoon," she said, "because that is when my fever comes to visit me and stays all night until the first light of day. My body then feels like when I was dancing, warm and sweaty, and my heart pounds. I used to be so afraid when it happened, but now it makes me sleepy. I fall into a deep peaceful sleep and dream. Oh, do I dream! I dream I am dancing on top of the mountain in the cool air, and everything smells good, instead of like disinfectant."

The nurse came into the room carrying a tray with a thermometer and jelly. "Well, I am glad to see you getting on so well with Gabrielle. Turn over, my little ballerina, time for your afternoon forecast. Doctor, you can step outside and have a smoke or something."

"Will you come back?" she asked.

"Of course, but I will have to take the five o'clock train."

From outside the door I could hear Gabrielle's gentle voice. "Can't you warm it up once? Why do you have to stick it in there? You know it will be high. Put it under my armpit. It is just as accurate."

"Gabrielle, the doctor wants a rectal temperature." Five minutes later the nurse was finished; she gave me a sad, knowing look and showed me the clipboard with the temperature record.

"What was it?" Gabrielle asked. "No, wait, let me guess— 104. Right? I can tell because I am becoming drowsy."

"Here, take two aspirins with a little water and you will cool down."

"And I will sweat and you will have to return to change all the sheets. If you didn't bother taking the temperature, Beatrice, I wouldn't need aspirins and you wouldn't have to change me."

"And the professor will send me out to take care of the cows," the nurse said.

"When you are ready to examine her Doctor, push this bell, and I will assist you."

"Thank you, but I still have to finish the history."

"Oh good," Gabrielle said cheerfully, "then you will have to return tomorrow and I will be all fresh and cleaned." The nurse placed a small glass filled with a purple solution on her night table.

"It is theophylline," the nurse said to me. "You take it, Gabrielle, and don't spill it out in the bathroom. You know it helps your wheezing. Doctor, see to it she drinks it. It opens her bronchial tubes."

"I hate it. What good is it. I drink it and then it only works for a few hours and I wheeze again."

"Gabrielle, would you prefer a suppository?"

"I will drink the purple poison, thank you."

She folded her milk-white slender arms in front of her and said, "Well go ahead, ask me questions."

The nurse left the room, and I placed my notebook on my lap. Before her eyes were cool and youthful-looking; now they were partially closed and wet. Her body was burning up from the fever. She had small narrow eyebrows that curved gently above her drooping eyelids, as if someone had sketched them in.

"Where were you born?"

"In the Valais, in Sion. Have you ever been there?"

"No."

"Then you must visit it before you return to New York."

"How do you know I am from New York?"

"Because I guessed. I know of three cities in America—New York, Chicago, Hollywood."

"Well, you are right, I am from New York. For a minute I thought you could tell from my New York accent. Did you have any childhood diseases?" I continued.

"Yes, scarletina, mumps, chicken pox, and something else that made my cough sound like a horn, not like the kind I have now."

"Whooping cough?"

"That's it."

I glanced at my watch and it was almost five. "I have to go, Gabrielle, because I will miss my train."

"Come tomorrow after breakfast. My room number is 26, so don't get lost. There are many Gabrielle's staying at Leysin, and you will have to start right from the beginning, introduce yourself and all that. And they won't be as patient as I."

"I will remember the number. Have a good night's rest."

"Can you open the window a little before you leave so then I can hear your train leave? I love to hear the train; it gives me hope that someday I will be on that train. Here in Leysin we live by sounds and light and smell, because the mountains are always the same. It is the lights that make it different. These mountains are my cell keepers, but the sounds of the train are the sounds of hope."

As I closed her door I felt a sad indescribable pain in my chest. The train back to Lausanne was crowded with medical students, nurses, and doctors who were free for the evening. As anxious as they were to leave for the city, so I yearned to stay with Gabrielle to look after her. What if she wheezed and coughed bitterly at night, and there was no one to hear? Being isolated like a punished child in a miserable dreary room was bad medical care. She only had a bell in her room to ring for help, but that was hundreds of yards away from the nurse's station.

Next to me on the train sat a student from Zurich who was also in his senior year. His speciality was going to be TB and respiratory diseases. "How do you like our Leysin?" he asked in English.

"I find it fascinating and sad."

"We give them excellent care and most of our patients recover. Dr. Jacquet's treatment has been successful for ninety percent of our in-patients. Our sanatorium has the best record in Europe. It is even better than your famous one in Saratoga. What part of the sanatorium are you visiting?"

I told him about my first encounter with Madame Corot and Gabrielle.

"Gabrielle is one of our more serious cases."

"Will she die?"

"She has not responded to Jacquet's treatment as well as we hoped, at least not yet."

I spent the remainder of the evening in the quiet of my room reading everything I could find on TB. The signs of worsening TB are a persistent fever, continual weight loss, gross spitting up of blood, and the TB lung cavity not shrinking. As I read, the image of Gabrielle's innocent red-cheeked face seemed to fill the page and I could hear her wheezing. Later I had a fretful sleep.

At seven o'clock the next morning I was back on the train to Leysin. I was the only medical student on board, along with the nurses and doctors and other helpers. The chief of the TB service approached me in the hall of the sanatorium.

"Do you Americans always start your day so early? The lectures will not begin until nine. Come and have some coffee with me."

"I need an earlier start because I haven't really finished my work from yesterday."

"Well, that is noble of you. Our Swiss students know they have all the time in the world. Some wait for years before they present themselves for the final doctorate examination. This is our system. I know in America there is no such laxity."

It was the end of November and the mountain air was damp. The clouds hung over the mountains like white curtains.

Ward B was deserted except for two orderlies pushing a stretcher with a body covered by a white sheet. I stopped short and wanted to pick up the sheet. Instead I rushed to Room 26 and found the door slightly ajar. With my hand I slowly pushed the door open, and with great joy and relief, I saw Gabrielle sitting up in bed reading a book of poems by Verlaine.

"Bon jour," I rejoiced.

"Aren't you a little early?" she said.

"I like to get an early start."

Her face was pale, and her eyes today looked like blue transparent glass.

"How do you feel?" I asked, as I still was standing by the door waiting to be asked inside.

"My fever came as usual, but it didn't stay so long. I feel much better, stronger, but you can't examine me until I am cleaned up and the sheets are changed. Come back at ten. But it is nice to see you so early. I expected you on the second train."

She looked remarkably better to me. "I guess Dr. Jacquet's treatment is beginning to work," she said with a smile.

"Then a little later I will return," and I closed the door behind me and bumped into the morning nurse who said sarcastically, "You might as well have stayed over."

My face became crimson as I scurried away from Ward B to see Madame Corot. Two women carrying the same illness;

the older one in stable condition, and then Gabrielle, desperately ill. That was the instructor's intent—to demonstrate the range of TB in 1952.

Madame Corot was in her chair where I had left her the day before. "Good morning Doctor," she said. "You are an early riser. That is good; it shows a strong character and devotion. I, too, have been up early. I have already taken my morning walk. A half-hour walk followed by a glass of fresh orange juice and then yogurt with fruit, emental with bread, and three vitamin pills. Last night I slept on my balcony for two hours in the cold air, which was invigorating, youthful. Did you ever read Boccaccio, Doctor, *The Nightingale?* You should. Then you could understand how I felt last night outside."

"Does Dr. Jacquet include champagne in his treatment program?" I asked in all seriousness.

"No, but he believes if the mind is well then cure is inevitable, and if a glass or two of champagne makes patients happy, he allows it. The professor believes the TB bacilli does not like good champagne, but the brain does. Do you know his theory, why people catch TB?"

"I don't," I said. "He has not lectured to us yet. Actually, I never met him."

"Oh, you will. If you don't meet him I will introduce you. He is a remarkable man. Not only is he a great doctor, but he is a major in the Swiss army. Now, to his theory: he believes people who have had terrible disappointments and who suffer from melancholy will develop TB or other diseases.

"My illness started when I was a young woman living at the palace where I worked as a private secretary to the sultan. My husband took up with the governess of one of the royalties and ran away with her, leaving me with a six-year-old child. I became so depressed that I planned to kill myself. At the palace they tried all sorts of potions and hydrobath cures. They soaked me in ice water and then put me into a steaming bath. The doctor of the palace was convinced that I had to be isolated from the palace. They placed me in a cell-like room, on a water diet with vitamins. I began to lose weight and still was dreadfully depressed. As I was all alone with no man in the prime of my youth, the wise man concluded it was necessary for me to have an operation to remove the excitable part of my body, the circumcision, as they called it. They removed my clitoris in one quick swipe of the razor while they administered ether."

"Where was this done?" I asked in a state of disbelief.

"At the palace there was a women's clinic for deliveries and other operations."

I remember reading that this type of barbaric treatment of women still existed even in 1950 in the Sudan, Kenya, and parts of West Africa. Circumcision of women was prescribed by Mohammedan law. Even in modern Egypt this operation was still performed on peasant girls.

"But this, too, did not cure my depression. And when I began to lose more weight and develop night sweats and started to cough blood, they diagnosed me as having tuberculosis and then sent me here to Leysin twenty-five years ago. You see, my young friend of twenty or so, the TB bacilli likes to live inside of unhappy people," she continued. "But you will learn about all of this while you are here. Even in so many of our famous stories, the heroine dies of TB from a lost love, like *Manon*. I became ill because of my misfortunes."

I wasn't convinced then or to this day that an illness could be caused or cured by the state of the mind alone. It is cured by a brilliant, marvelous drug that kills the bacilli. Antibiotics for TB, when they were discovered, closed all the sanatoriums in a few years as they cured the patients. So it was with every illness we have had, and today, AIDS and cancer will have to be cured with the magic bullet, once it is found, and not just by thinking good thoughts.

The nurse arrived one hour later and Madame Corot was undressed and put into a hospital gown. I examined her lungs, heart, and stomach, and when I was finished I had found no abnormalities.

"Well Doctor—what then should I call a second-year medical student?—you found nothing. I am glad; it means I am getting better."

I thanked her for allowing me to examine her and then proceeded to the lecture hall where Jacquet was to give his talk. As on the first morning, he never arrived, instead his assistant described the terminal aspect of TB.

The X-ray department was located on the ground floor and was attended by a Russian doctor called Boris Babiantz. I found Madame Corot's chest X rays, and then hand-carried them to the reading room where Professor Babiantz was sipping coffee and smoking a cigarette.

"We haven't taken a film from Madame Corot in years," he said. "She refuses to be X-rayed. This one was taken five years ago," he said.

We both looked at her films—he with his expert eye and I as a novice. "Are you sure these are her films?" he asked.

"This is what they gave me."

"According to these films, she no longer has active TB," he said. "In essence, she is cured. We perform X rays on the patients once every six months. There must be other films on file."

We looked through the old files in the basement and did locate her chest films from ten years earlier, which demonstrated the classical TB signs, a large hole, or a cavity, in the lung.

"How does she feel?" the radiologist asked.

"She complains of fatigue, but I did not find anything on the examination."

"Well then, ask the doctor in charge of her case to order some sputum collections. The TB bacilli is found in the sputum, and in some cases even in the urine. According to the number of TB in the sputum, the TB is classified as to its infectability as $1+$ to $4+$. The latter indicates a marked contagious stage, and then extra precautions are taken by the staff."

At this sanatorium there seemed to be no signs of anyone taking precautions, such as wearing masks and gloves when examining the patients. At the beginning of each stay at Leysin the students had a skin test for TB and a fluoroscopic examination of their lungs, which was then repeated again before they left. Most of the doctors who stayed at Leysin developed a positive test for TB. A positive test meant that a mild form of TB had been contracted.

As I was leaving the X-ray department to return to see Madame Corot, I met Dr. Jacquet. His bald head looked like a shiny bowling ball set with two large dark eyes that looked like onyx stones. He was a small man, but with large powerful arms and legs. And when he shook hands with me I could hear my fingers crack from his solid grip.

"I hope you will enjoy your stay here in Leysin," he said slowly in English. "My office is open to you if you have any questions or problems." With that he disappeared, like Peter Rabbit scurrying into the hall. I never saw him again for the rest of my stay in Leysin.

It was eleven o'clock in the morning when I returned to visit with Madame Corot. The sun still had not broken through the clouds and the mountains were not visible. There was the dampness in the air before it begins to snow. She was sitting on her chaise longue on the balcony, wearing sunglasses even though there was no sun.

"The lights up here are very strong," she said, "that they hurt my eyes." She was wearing a Persian lamb fur coat and a Persian hat, looking like a Russian princess riding on a sled.

"I am sorry to bother you again."

"This is no bother," she answered. "What else is there for me to do?"

"I want to ask you some more questions before I write up your report."

"I know about the report, how important it is for the students. You are very serious. Relax a little, young man. You will be all worn out before you are thirty. You must save some of your energies for the better things in life, if you know what I mean. Well, go on then, ask some more questions."

In the European medical school system there were no examinations until the end of the year, and most of the learning was left up to the student, except for the medical reports that, it was rumored, the professors never read.

I asked Madame Corot again the same questions.

"As I told you doctor, I am only tired, and if I do just what the doctor tells me, I get by each day. It is almost lunch. Can I offer you a glass of Moët? I have had enough of the balcony for now, and I must write some correspondence before lunch because the mail leaves at three."

I was glad the interview was over because it was raw outside, and I felt my bones shake from the cold air. Or was it from her dark Turkish eyes piercing me?

Dr. Duvalle was the immediate doctor in charge of Madame Corot. He was a man about fifty years old with gray hair growing out of his nose. He had an expression on his face as if he were always smelling something foul. His lips were curled up towards his nose. We barely exchanged greetings, and when I asked about collecting sputums from Madame Corot, he gave me an annoying look and said, "When you write your report, include that as part of the suggestions," he said.

"But would it not be better if I had the sputum results so I can write a thorough report, including the prognosis?"

"Your 'stage' will be finished in a week or so, and it takes several months for the culture. Unless, of course, you would like to stay here for the rest of the semester and wait for the cultures to return in two months?

"Oh, by the way, it is not necessary for you to arrive here at seven in the morning unless you want to help in the kitchen to prepare breakfast."

He was an obnoxious doctor, and I would be meeting many more like him in the future. How can such an insensitive man work with patients? I wondered. But when one of the patients strolled past him, he was remarkably charming and warm. He transformed into a different person—the doctor was not the same person as the man who had told me to become kitchen help.

After lunch I was on the large terrace, which looked like a deck of a luxury ocean liner. Although there was no sun, and the sky was covered with great ominous clouds, the patients were lying on chaise longues, barely dressed, taking their out-door cure. I was shivering from the damp air, but the patients tolerated the cold better than I.

Gabrielle was lying on one of those chairs, covered with a light sheet, still reading her book of poetry. For a few minutes I watched her from a distance. Her long brown hair came down to her shoulders, and her face had a peaceful look. She was the youngest one on the terrace today. Occasionally, she looked up, giving a pleasant greeting to a passerby.

"Hello, Gabrielle. Aren't you cold?"

"A little, but I get used to it. Dr. Jacquet said it is the best thing for me. I missed you this morning. I was all cleaned up, waiting for you to examine me."

"I know. I am sorry. I had to see another patient."

"Was she pretty?"

"Yes, but not as pretty as you. She is old enough to be your grandmother," I said.

"Pull a chair over and sit a little while with me. Then we can go in, and you can examine me. You are wearing a different tie today," she said.

I had not noticed it. I just grabbed any tie because I rushed out to the train.

"You are as old as I am, I bet," she said.

"Just about; perhaps a year or two older."

"Do you have a girlfriend in America?"

"No."

"How about here in Lausanne?"

"No, Gabrielle. I have no girlfriends. I am too busy to find a girlfriend."

"You are a cute-looking guy. I bet there are plenty of girls who would like to go out with an American medical student."

"Well, I have not met them yet."

"Do you like to dance?"

"No, I don't know how to very well."

"I could teach you when I get better. I would like to dance for you."

"I would be honored, Gabrielle."

"It will take me a long time to get back into shape. Ballet is really hard work." She moved her small body under the sheet as if she were standing by an exercise bar in front of a mirror.

"I dance *Petrouchka* the best, and *Swan Lake*. Have you ever seen a ballet?"

"Yes, I saw *Swan Lake* in New York, and the *Nutcracker Suite*."

"I was invited to the Metropolitan Ballet School for one year, but then I became ill," she said softly. Her eyes became moist, and I felt a sick feeling in the pit of my stomach.

"Can you take me back to my cell," she said. "I am getting chilled. I think the fever is coming back."

I wheeled her back to the room under the suspicious eyes of the other patients.

"Now, if the other doctors were as thoughtful," teased the nurse from the morning, whose name was Nurse Marais, "it would make our work easier."

"Can you help me? I have to examine Gabrielle for my write-up."

"It is not necessary," Gabrielle said.

"It is a hospital rule, Gabrielle. No doctor examines a female patient without a nurse, especially young, handsome, male medical students."

The nurse gave me a knowing glance. Nurse Marais had that mature look of an understanding woman. She was a large woman who reminded me of the actress Simone Signoret. It was obvious she cared a great deal about the gentle Gabrielle, not only as a patient but as if she were her daughter.

I waited outside the door as Gabrielle was undressed and made ready for the examination. "Come on in, doctor of the future," I heard Nurse Marais yell. "I just took her temperature for you, Doctor, and it is normal for the first time in weeks. You bring good luck to Gabrielle."

I looked into her mouth first and found her tonsils to be small, but not infected. I examined her tiny ears with an otoscope, and I could hear her breathing close to my ear. Nurse Marais undid her hospital gown and held it in front of her chest as I proceeded to examine her lungs. I tapped the back of her chest to find areas of dullness and areas that would sound like a drum if there were a cavity underneath my hand. I could not find any of these abnormalities until Gabrielle said, "You have to go higher. That is where my cavity lies. Here," she said, and twisted her hand in back, touching my hand.

She was right. The tapping sound changed dramatically to a sound like a drummer playing. With my hand flat on her chest, I asked her to whisper "33," which would give me a clue if the lungs were filled with fluid or contained a cavity. My stethoscope on her chest moved slowly each inch as I heard both lungs wheeze and rattle and gurgle like a sulfur geyser I had once heard on a volcanic mountain. I moved to the front of her chest and Nurse Marais dropped the sheet, revealing her youthful body. Gabrielle's face flushed, and she closed her eyes as I listened to her heart.

Before the invention of the stethoscope in the 1800s, doctors placed their ears directly on the patient's chest. Besides causing all sorts of embarrassing problems for the female patients and doctors, there was also the fear of catching fleas from the patient, which was what prompted the great youthful clinician Laennec of France to remedy the situation by the invention of the stethoscope. All of Europe made a mockery of Laennec's "tube" for almost fifty years. The American Supreme Court Justice Oliver Wendell Holmes even wrote a humorous poem about Laennec's stethoscope.

In Leysin the older doctors, on occasion, still placed their ear directly on the chest for better hearing of the sounds of the heart and lungs.

The front of her chest was wheezing as loud as the back, and her heart was racing. Her eyes opened, and she looked directly at me as I listened to her heart under her breast. I felt my face turn beet red and swiftly moved away as Nurse Marais recovered her moist chest.

She started to wheeze more than ever, and Nurse Marsais poured some theophylline into a glass which Gabrielle swiftly drank. "Do you make all your patients wheeze?" the nurse joked.

"Only if they are allergic to me," I quickly replied.

"Very clever, doctor."

Gabrielle was now lying on the pillow. Her face had turned a purple-red, but her wheezing had subsided to some degree.

"I am very sick and am I not . . ." she said with a sad, desperate voice.

"Not so sick, Gabrielle. I have seen others who are much sicker and get better and cured."

"You better learn to lie so it doesn't show on your face, because no patient will believe what you say."

"Look, Gabrielle, I am only a medical student. You are my second case of TB. I have examined you and you ask me questions like I was some kind of expert. I really don't know how sick you are."

"Don't get annoyed. I was only trying to get information."

"I am not annoyed, just frustrated."

"Well, then you need a girlfriend."

Nurse Marais gleamed with pleasure as we carried on this way. She reminded me that the last train was leaving in minutes.

"Are you coming early again, before the rest of the students?" Gabrielle asked.

"Of course I am. I have to look at your X ray and write up your report and that of the other patient I examined. Well, have a good evening."

"I will miss you until tomorrow."

I wanted to tell her I would miss her too, but I dared not.

Nurse Marais accompanied me down the long hall and said, "You did very well. She is very sick, the poor sweetheart, and she cares a lot for you."

"And I for her," I said.

"When is your stage over?"

"In a few days," I told her.

"Don't tell her unless she asks. She has no friends here and does not get many visitors, except once a month her parents come. She is so young and beautiful," the nurse continued, "and she is a dreamer. She resents the doctors and all the people who can come and go freely. I am always afraid she will do something foolish."

"Like what?" I asked in panic.

"Like leaving her bed at night and walking to the edge of the terrace and throwing herself down the mountain."

"But that can't be possible. She has to be watched then all the time."

"That is not possible."

"Has it happened?"

"Yes, but they are usually older ones who take the stroll to the bottom."

Back in the city that night I wrote up the case of Madame Corot while I kept thinking about Gabrielle. It was a long ten-page report, and my conclusion was that Madame Corot no longer had active TB and could be discharged from the sanatorium at any time.

The following morning I chose a bright red tie and blue shirt and took extra time to comb my hair. I brought a bouquet of white flowers for Gabrielle. The sky was cold and gray when I arrived at the top of the mountain. This morning the hospital looked deserted. Then I realized it was Saturday and most of the students and staff would be off until Monday morning.

Gabrielle was sleeping peacefully and her face looked angelic with some beads of perspiration on her white forehead. Sleep is a blessing for the sick; it is the only refuge they have from the horror of the reality of their illness.

Dr. Duvalle, the obnoxious doctor of the floor, greeted me coldly as I arrived on Ward B. "I finished my report on Madame Corot," I told him.

"That is very good. Leave it on my desk and I will grade it and return it to you on Monday. What is your conclusion?" he asked.

"I think she no longer has active TB."

"You are likely correct. Why don't you tell her the good news. She will be most grateful to you, and then she can leave, and Dr. Jacquet can chalk up another cure."

Madame Corot was sitting at her table in the center of the room. The table was covered with a gold brocaded Ottoman rug, and she was sipping coffee from a small cup.

"Will you have some real Turkish coffee?" she asked. "On Saturday, I treat myself with this luxury. You are an enthusiastic young man. Have you come to examine me again?"

"Well, I came to tell you some great news about your illness."

"I always like to hear good news. What is it?"

"I spoke to the doctor, Duvalle."

"He is not my doctor. My personal doctor is Dr. Jacquet. Anyway, go on."

"You no longer have TB, and you can leave the sanatorium."

"Are you sure?"

"Well, I think so. Dr. Duvalle agrees. I wanted to tell you the first thing in the morning. I was so excited."

She remained silent and quietly sipped her coffee. "Where is your report now?" she asked. "I would like to see it."

"It is in Dr. Duvalle's office."

She slowly moved up from her chair, faced the icon on her night table, and placed her hands together as if to pray. "You fool," she started quietly and then began to scream. "This is my home. I can't leave here. Where will I go? I have no home like you. I have been here for twenty-five years, and you tell me I am cured. How dare you say that. Dr. Jacquet knows I am still sick. I can't go out there. Please leave this room and never return. I can't leave here until I die!" she screamed and began to sob like I had never heard a person cry so desperately before.

Dr. Duvalle had heard the screaming from the room and was at the door when I left.

"What happened in there?" he asked. He saw my pale face and smirked with delight.

"I told her she was cured. Why didn't you tell me I shouldn't."

"You didn't ask."

"You knew all this time she did not have to be here?"

"Yes. We sort of let her stay here and go along with her madness, but now it will have to change."

"Why?"

"Because she will have to come to our weekly conference on whom can be discharged. You will be back in Lausanne completing your studies and get a wonderful recommendation for your thorough work, and she will be out on the street."

"That is insane. Why blame it on me? You assigned me to the case."

"Unless of course, you want to withdraw your report, and you will get an incomplete."

"I am not going to hold back on the truth," I yelled at him.

"That is your choice, sir."

This was my first lesson on the mystique of the practice of medicine. As I have learned over and over again, some people will never forgive you for trying to help or even save their lives. Madame Corot was using her illness to keep a roof over her head. I later learned that her stay at Leysin would be paid for as long as she remained. It was her choice to make this her life home. Actually, the doctors were being humanitarians by going along with her madness. Or had they been doing her a great disservice by not having forced her back to the mainstream of life years ago?

The radiologist on call for the weekend was well acquainted with Gabrielle's illness. He swiftly retrieved her X-ray films, and in the darkness of the room he uttered a sad sigh.

"If you look here, she has two large TB cavities which are not healing. That corresponds to your physical findings," the doctor said. "We collapsed the lung once, called a pneumothorax, which did nothing to help her. Medical treatment is a continual game of hit and misses, luckily most patients get better despite their treatment."

He saw the forlorn look on my face in the darkness of the X-ray room. He offered me a cigarette. "It doesn't look good for her."

"So you think she will die?"

"I am not a medical doctor, just a radiologist. My life is lived in the shadows of the day and I deal in shadows. That is the question you have to address to Dr. Jacquet when he returns. Some patients live on for months, others for weeks, and then there is always the chance a cure for TB will be developed. They are not too far from it now. There is a doctor by the name of Waxman, in Boston, who has been working on such a drug.

"You have a special interest in this case?" he asked me.

"I care a lot for Gabrielle. She is too young to die."

"We all do. She is as gentle as an edelweis flower on our mountains. Her sputum is swarming with active TB bacilli." the radiologist continued. "She also has a heart murmur that has developed since she's been in the hospital."

"A heart murmur? I did not hear one. I examined her just yesterday."

"It is not easy to hear. One of our interns picked it up and the cardiologist confirmed it. That is another one of her problems we have to solve. She doesn't have rheumatic fever, which is so common today in our young people, and the heart murmur is getting louder."

This was not a good day for me. First I caused great chaos

in Madame Corot's life, and now I had completely missed a heart murmur. In my write-up of Gabrielle's case, I would have flunked miserably if I had failed to find the murmur.

"Go and listen to her heart again and you will hear it. That is why you go to medical school, to learn. Don't look so downcast. This won't be the first time you will miss a heart murmur. Why do you think I became a radiologist?" he laughed. He placed his arm about my shoulder and again said, "You can only become a doctor if you care and if you experience failure. It makes you humble and more careful. It is not the end of the world."

Gabrielle was sitting up in a chair by the window, her hair now tied in a pony tail with a small red ribbon. "Thank you for the paper narcissus. They are beautiful."

"How are you feeling?"

"Better, but a little sad. Look outside." The entire world outside was painted white. The mountains were no longer visible and the last few red autumn leaves were now off the trees. It was snowing heavily, like in the heart of winter.

"Snow comes early to Leysin and never leaves," she said. "Professor Jacquet makes us lie out on the snow when the sun is out with only our underclothing on."

"Gabrielle, I have to listen to your heart again."

"How nice. You know it makes me a little nervous, but only when you examine me. I love your bedside manners. You are so gentle."

"I am going to call the nurse. I will be right back."

"You don't have to call the nurse. I trust you."

"I'd rather call the nurse, Gabrielle."

Nurse Marais, luckily, was working the weekend. She was sitting at her desk, busy writing in the charts.

"I am sorry to bother you, but could you help me again. I have to listen to Gabrielle's heart."

"You did already, yesterday."

"I know, but I missed a heart murmur completely. I can't write the report up until I hear it."

"It is Saturday. All the students are gone. Why don't you go back to Lausanne? Come back on Monday. I am the only nurse on for two wings." She looked as me again. "When you get that puppy look on your face," she said, "you and that little ballerina, I can't resist. All right, come on. You have ten minutes."

"I need five."

This time I listened to Gabrielle's heart first while she was sitting up and then lying down, and the murmur was there. It came from one of the valves of the heart, but I was not certain from which one.

"Why are you listening so much? Do I have heart trouble now? If I do, it is all your fault."

"Thank you, Nurse Marais," I said.

"Will you be back today?" Gabrielle asked.

"Yes, but I have to write up your case before I forget everything."

There was a large comfortable library with easy chairs, tables, and good lighting. I described my findings in detail and wrote my conclusions, which troubled me because my only diagnosis was pulmonary TB; I still was left without an explanation for the cause of the heart murmur.

It was past five P.M. when I finally finished the long write-up, and it was dark outside. The snow fell furiously with wind howling circles around the sanatorium.

When I returned to Gabrielle's room the nurse told me the trains would not be running until the morning because of the storm.

"Oh, wonderful. Then you will have to stay here all night. Thank you, storm," Gabrielle said.

"I suppose you will want to eat here with the princess," the nurse said.

With not much resolution I said, "I will eat in the cafeteria."

"I will bring you a tray, too, and perhaps through some sniffing around I can find a carafe of wine. You worked hard today and you deserve it. But don't go shouting this to the other students because then there will be trouble."

One half-hour later, Nurse Marais brought two trays, a small white tablecloth, and two candles with a carafe of red wine.

"There now, my *petite, bon appetit.*" She returned minutes later with a blanket and a pillow. "In case you decide to sleep on the chair next to mademoiselle."

There was a small radio in the room and Edith Piaf was singing, *"Mon Homme,"* my man.

"Do you like the Little Bird too?" Gabrielle asked.

"She is my favorite singer," I replied.

I lit the two small candles on the round table and ate the usually unappetizing hospital meal, but which tonight was like a feast. The candlelight's glow made Gabrielle's face appear languid and beautiful. We ate the small pieces of ripened Camembert while sipping on the wine for dessert. Gabrielle's face turned red. At first I thought it was the wine, but it was her night temperature rising. She tried to suppress a cough, and then her wheezing became audible in the room. She rose from the table and opened the drab-looking blinds.

"I have to open the window just a bit. It helps me breathe better."

Snowflakes settled on her brown hair as they sped through the window. She took a swallow of the purple medicine by her bedside and the wheezing began to subside. From her dresser she brought out some photographs of herself and placed them on the table like a fortune player.

"Perhaps it will be the worst snowstorm of the century, and you will have to stay here for days with me. Would you like that?"

"Yes, I would like that very much."

"These are my parents in front of our house, and my two sisters."

"They all look like you," I remarked, "not as pretty."

"Do you think I am pretty."

"Of course, very."

"Much prettier than any of your girlfriends."

"Yes, if I had any girlfriends."

"Then you really like me?"

"Yes, of course I do. I like you a lot, Gabrielle."

She gave me a sweet coy smile and loosened the little ribbon which held her hair. It came falling down to her back as gently as the snowflakes were falling outside.

"This is me dancing." She produced a photograph of herself doing a pirouette, wearing her leotards. Other photographs followed, showing Gabrielle in her *Petrushka* costume. She looked at the photographs with an anguished expression on her face.

"I will never dance again," she said in a solemn voice. "You saw my X ray, did you not?"

"Yes."

"Well, they must be pretty bad. When do you think I will die?"

"That is ridiculous! You don't know what you are saying. If you are going to talk like that I am going to leave."

She started to cry. I wanted to cry with her. I sat next to her and placed my arms around her small soft shoulders.

"You did that to get my sympathy Gabrielle, and it won't work. You will be cured in a few months and you won't even remember me when you get back to your stage life."

"Then I will be all right. Are you sure? I believe you for tonight. Because tonight is a magical night. I feel so alive for the first time since I came to Leysin. God sent the snow to keep you here for me. I want to dance for you."

"I want to see you dance, which will be very soon."

"Not very soon. Now. Tonight. I feel strong enough. You step outside and I will put on my leotards. Return in a few minutes. Dr. Jacquet said that some exercise is good for me."

"Gabrielle, you can't dance now. You are not strong enough. You might harm yourself." She started to undo her robe. "All right. All right. Call when you are ready."

When I returned she was dressed in her leotards, and she looked adorable. Her hair was now drawn into a bun, and she stood bent over slightly with her delicate arms crossed over her side. Slowly she moved her body gracefully, with her arms stretched, circling in mid-air, and then she was on her toes circling the room, then jumping in the air as I stood entranced by this strange scene. For a moment we were both transported to a recital hall. Beads of perspiration appeared on her forehead as she bounced from one end of the small room to the other. Her eyes always focused on me. Then she stopped, bowed her head and knelt down as I applauded.

"That was beautiful, Gabrielle. You are incredible."

"Did you really like me?"

"Yes, I'm speechless."

She fell back on the bed, wiping her forehead with a towel.

"Now I am tired. I want to take a little rest, but you now have to read to me with your cute French accent from my poetry book. Here," she said, "read *The Living Flame* by Baudelaire. I will close my eyes and imagine we are in a small café in Paris on the left bank, and we are sipping on fine cognac and coffee and it is late at night."

I started to read the beautiful poem out loud. One of the lines I was fearful to recite: "They sing of Death, you sing the Resurrection; ... Bright stars whose brilliance no sun can dull!"

Gabrielle was sleeping soundly and I covered her perspiring

body with a blanket. I sat in the hard, uncomfortable chair, scrutinizing her labored breathing. This was the first of many more times to come when I would be sitting by the bedside of a critically ill patient. Sweet Gabrielle, so young and innocent. Why should she be suffering so much? I could not imagine the world without Gabrielle.

Several hours later she awoke, uttering a soft gentle sigh, as if she were returning from a beautiful dream. I was sitting in the chair finishing up her case history.

"You are still here while I am sleeping. I am sorry. You must be so bored."

"Actually not, I was doing my homework."

"Writing about me? I hope it is nice things." She pulled the vase of flowers from her night table and held them close to her bosom.

"These are so beautiful. No one ever gave me flowers like this. Now I know you like me a little."

She sat up and her face blushed. "I never had a man, and I am going to die, no matter what you say. Do you like me a lot?"

"Yes, you know I do."

"Do you think I am sexy? You did see me when you examined me."

"I remember well."

"Well?"

"Well what? You are a beautiful young woman."

"Do you like my body?"

"Gabby, that is not a question to ask."

"You called me Gabby. No one ever called me that."

"In America, you would be called Gabby."

"Will you do one thing for me tonight, because tonight is my night? It was given to us."

I feared what was coming next.

"Make love to me. You don't have to kiss me, just touch me. I just want to know how it feels. I dreamed you did. It was such a heavenly dream. No one would know, and I would not betray you. You don't have to kiss me, because my mouth is filled with the deadly bacteria, and I wouldn't want you to get sick. You are too sweet and dear to me."

I wanted to race to her and place my arms around her to protect from the angel of death, but she saw the anguish on my face and began to cry, "I am sorry." She cried herself to sleep while I sat motionless and confused on the chair, not knowing what to do.

When early morning finally arrived, I silently crept out of the room as she remained in her peaceful sleep. The trains were running again. Outside it was still dark. It stopped snowing and a sliver of moonlight reflected on the white night. The snow was as pure as the young woman I had left. I did not need Hippocrates's oath to convince me how I had to behave at that enticing moment, and my vulnerability would be many times tested during my medical career. Falling in love with a patient is one thing, but to take advantage of a woman who confides all her trust in a doctor is despicable. I wanted to maintain the doctor-patient relationship with Gabrielle and act as her healer rather than her lover, lest she lose all respect for me.

I watched the sun rise over the Alps from the train, which moved slowly throught the snow-packed tracks. When I arrived back at my small room in the hotel where I was staying, I had decided that I was going to care for Gabrielle. This was the first time I had ever felt so deeply about someone. I would speak to the chief of the service to get permission to see her every weekend until she was well, not as a student but as her friend.

I spent Sunday in the library and then searched for a present I would give her on Monday morning. All the stores were closed except a tobacconist, and I found a funny-looking cow-boy made of marzipan.

On Monday morning I took the five o'clock train to Leysin. My heart was pounding with anticipation of seeing my ballet dancer. I waited for the freight elevator, which finally arrived. There was a body in the elevator on a stretcher pushed by two orderlies. The Monday morning transferring of the dead. When I arrived at Ward B there was no one on the floor. The hall smelled of oxalic acid disinfectant. Gabrielle's door was opened and inside a woman was kneeling on the floor with a pail, scrubbing the walls. The bed was empty.

I raced outside, looking for the nurse or doctor. There was an older man and a woman standing by the nurses's desk. I recognized them from the pictures that Gabrielle had shown me. They were her parents signing some papers, and they were given a bag of clothing.

"Where is Gabrielle? What happened?"

"Gabrielle is in heaven," the woman said and started to cry.

"She died on Sunday," Nurse Marais softly said. "She died in her sleep."

I looked at her parents and felt I had known them all my life. Her mother had the same face as Gabrielle.

"Did you know my daughter?" the father asked.

"Yes, we were friends for a short time."

I had to look away because tears filled my eyes.

In the following weeks, streptomycin was introduced for the treatment of TB in Boston—the miracle drug that arrived too late to save Gabrielle. I never returned to Leysin again. In spite of my medical report, which I had submitted, Madame Corot was permitted to stay until the sanatorium closed, for the new treatment of TB had cured most of the patients.

Many weeks later I found the picture of Gabrielle in her

leotards on the inside of my jacket pocket. She must have slipped it into my pocket while I fell asleep at her bedside. It had a small inscription written, "This is how I want you to remember me," and she quoted one other line of the poem we had read together: "You sing the Resurrection of my soul."

NINE

Night Train to Paris

"THERE IS A robber on the train!" an imp of a man was shouting, racing through our train compartment. "Hide your money! He has already stolen some."

I was on the night train from Venice to Paris. It was October 1978. The three other men in our first-class compartment quickly hid their wallets under the seats and stuffed their money into their socks and boots.

The three men were Italians from a small town in Sicily. The older man and his two sinister-looking sons were actually looking forward to meeting the robber—the long train ride had become terribly boring. The father, a small man, his face weathered from the hot Sicilian sun, sat quietly, smiling. His feet did not touch the ground and one of the sons had placed a well-travelled, battered suitcase on the floor so his father could rest his feet. The other son placed a blue pillow behind the wrinkled head and the old man smiled with gratitude. I returned his smile, saying, "This will be an exciting trip with a robber on the train."

"No English," he said, somewhat breathlessly.

"No Italian," I said.

He threw up his hands in disappointment. The older son gave him a magazine with many pictures. He held it between his worn hands. The magazine shook like a leaf in the wind, and I could hear labored breathing behind the glossy pages. Occasionally he chuckled gently, showed the pictures to his sons, which caused all of them to break out into convulsive laughter. The old man enjoyed touching the soft red velvet of the upholstered seat on which he sat like a Buddhist priest. He rubbed the material with his hand and smiled contentedly to himself.

My eyes found his feet resting on the valise. He wore small brown narrow shoes, and they looked even smaller than they were because his ankles were as swollen as baby balloons. He bent his tiny wrinkled head and whispered something to his sons. They swiftly and deftly lifted him off the soft seat and escorted him out to the toilet. With each step he gasped desperately to catch his breath. They returned ten minutes later, and by then he was coughing violently. Like a small child, they lifted him ever so gently onto the seat, and he gratefully fell back, exhausted from the walk. The violent coughing continued. The youngest son reached into his pocket and brought forth a small bottle that contained a purple solution. He poured it into a spoon, which he gingerly placed into the mouth of the old man. The color of the liquid told me it must be liquified digitalis. The poor man had congestive heart failure, and the sons were trying their best to help. All this time they never uttered a word to me, but frequently stared in my direction. Each time I tried to speak they stared directly into my eyes. The old man kept inadvertently shaking his head to and fro, up and down, like a puppet.

It was becoming very warm in the compartment, and I stood

up to open the window. The fresh air would be good for the old man. He needed oxygen and a strong diuretic to give him some relief. The oldest son jumped up and shook an admonishing finger at me, barking in Italian. I retreated without a word.

They removed the old man's jacket and unbuttoned his shirt collar, revealing two large pulsating veins on his neck, a sure sign of heart failure, especially when considered along with his swollen ankles. Gratefully, he gently took one of the son's hands, held it in his own, smiling. He had such a peaceful look on his face. I had seen this look before, from those about to die who have lived fully, taken care of all their affairs, and had no more unfinished details of life to distress them.

I wondered why they were traveling for so long with such a sick man on their hands. Perhaps there was a relative in Paris he wanted to see before he died.

When they had helped the old man to the toilet I had noticed that he was bent over, like a man searching for coins on the ground, and his ears stood out displaying blue cartilage. Both of his sons also had large curvatures of the spine, and they, too, had deep blue cartilage ears, as if someone had painted them for a carnival.

There is a disease, affecting members of the same family, which causes blue cartilage to show in ears and nose and blue coloration of the eyes. It is a strange disease called ochronosis, an error of metabolism that forces the beautiful blue pigment to accumulate in vital areas. It can cause heart failure and also affects the spine and bends the neck, like an ostrich's in the sand. Frequently mental retardation is a concomitant of the lovely shades of blue.

From the luggage rack above their heads, they brought down a basket of food and served the old man sausage and bread. The sausage was poison for the old man because there was enough salt in it to trap him in congestive heart failure until he died.

The younger man held a Spanish wine bag in his hand and squirted wine into his ugly mouth. Then the old man opened his mouth like a small nesting bird and waited for the wine to stream in. It missed the mark and his face was covered with wine, which made him laugh. The sons took out a dirty-looking rag and wiped the old man's face. The old man again whispered something into the ears of the older son, who shook his head to say no. "No food for the foreigner," they must have said. They watched me with the suspicion reserved for those from another time and place.

The younger son suddenly stalked out of the compartment, a tiger on the prowl, sniffing the air to detect if the robber was nearby. He glided through the long narrow passageway. The older son, who had rat eyes, leaned back in his seat, folded his arms and burped, suffusing the compartment with the overwhelming odor of digesting sausage.

The old man finally stopped coughing when the other son returned from the hunt leaving the compartment door open and perching on the very edge of his seat. He reached into his black leather jacket pocket and pulled out a long knife, which, until now, had been concealed in a small leather case. He held the stiletto affectionately, turning it in his rough hands, and then began to clean his nails. It seemed odd that he should have been so concerned about his nails because the rest of him was so unkempt. His trousers were spotted, as was the brown shirt opened at the collar.

The old man started coughing again—a dry, painful, rapid, hacking cough that sounded like the train as it sped over the tracks. He then removed a filthy handkerchief from somewhere in his baggy trousers and spat into it. It looked like blood-streaked saliva. If he did have TB, the compartment would now be swarming with TB bacilli.

The steward suddenly appeared, announcing that the first

sitting of dinner was about to take place. "Please lock up all your things. The robber has not been caught," he told us in French. The two sons, who must have understood enough, looked happily at each other.

I was relieved to leave the sick compartment and wondered if my traveling bags would still be there when I returned. I felt their eyes on my neck and heard the coughing of the old man echoing in my ears as I quickly moved down the train compartment to the dining room.

I asked the steward about changing compartments. "There is only a place in third class, sir," he said, "and you have to wait until the next stop at the border to change wagons."

With some trepidation, after prolonging my dinner, I returned to the same compartment. They were eating again, speaking among themselves as if I weren't there. The older son was using the same knife that he had used to clean his nails to cut the sausage. He passed the neatly sliced pieces to his father and brother who wolfed them down with bread. The older son held the wine bag in one hand and squeezed; the stream of blood-red wine poured into his mean-looking mouth.

I felt like I was intruding on their dinner and stepped out of the compartment. Darkness had set in, and the small villages that we passed were barely discernible. We passed through the Italian Alps, and I could see Lake Maggiore through the darkness. The Swiss border was nearly upon us, but there was still a twelve-hour ride to Paris.

Suddenly, I heard loud voices coming from another compartment, and then a young man with a ponytail ran past me, followed by an older woman in her nightgown screaming in English, "I have been robbed!"

The two brothers sprang from the compartment, the older with his knife in hand, his eyes blazing and expectant, like those of a wild animal. He took chase after the the robber.

Then there was a loud and terrifying scream. I feared to see what horror had been done, and I turned back to the compartment. The old man was sitting on his seat, his eyes popping. Minutes later the two brothers returned. The one with the knife was wiping it on his handkerchief, grinning. They whispered something to the old man, who began to laugh like a clown. Two train officials appeared and took statements from the brothers, who were looking proud because they had stopped the robber.

The old man looked on, waiting to hear the details from his sons, and then he began to cough again. His cough was now different from before. He gasped for air, and he began to froth at the mouth, like he was blowing bubbles. He suddenly fell back, his face turned red, then violet blue, and his lips puffed out like a blowfish. Doctors many times act by reflex. We are trained to save lives. Cardiac arrest is, alas, a familiar happening in my life as a cardiologist. Without a second thought, I leaped up from my seat and lurched towards the old man, punching him on the chest to try to resuscitate the heart that had stopped, yelling to the sons to breathe into his mouth.

"I am a cardiologist," I yelled as the sons angrily pushed me away. I tried reaching for him again, but as I raised my fist over his chest they began yelling at me in Italian and pummelling me in the head until I fell back.

"I am a doctor. I want to help him. Breathe into his mouth. We have to stimulate his heart."

I felt their hands around me like iron shackles and expected to feel the stiletto in my chest any second. The old man now lay motionless on the seat. His sons stared at me, fire blazing in their eyes.

"*Assassino!*" they yelled with tears in their red eyes as they pushed me down on the floor of the compartment and began kicking me in the head and sides. The more I resisted and screamed for help, the more I added fuel to their passion.

From outside the compartment I heard the steward, "Passports please," and then, just as the older brother was about to land his dirty boot on my skull, the Swiss border police rushed into the compartment and swiftly restrained the two madmen. I suffered minor injuries, but the humiliation of trying to save a life while almost giving up mine was much more painful to me than the pummelling by those men.

The train stopped at the Swiss border, and we were taken off the train, along with the dead body of the old man and that of the robber.

I explained to the Swiss police my efforts to resuscitate the old man.

A Swiss doctor came on the scene and pronounced the two men dead. He placed his hand on my shoulder, understanding the unpleasant circumstances, and sadly said, "People from the country have not heard of CPR yet," he said. "It's best not to interfere."

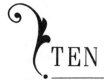

TEN

The Marquise of Toulouse

LITTLE DID I dream of the bizarre adventure that awaited me when I first met the Marquis and the Marquise of Toulouse. I was in medical school in Switzerland, and I had decided to spend one month in Toulouse with a great professor, Jean Riviere, the famed diagnostician. I stayed in a small hotel called the Henry IV along with three other Americans who were Fulbright students. The Marquis and Marquise of Toulouse learned of our arrival and wasted no time in contacting us, wishing to improve their English by conversing with American students.

The Marquise arrived in her chauffeured limousine on a brisk clear October evening. She was taking us to dinner at her chateau. We all met in the small foyer of the hotel when she suddenly appeared, a beautiful woman in a long black dress. The chauffeur introduced us: "This is the Marquise of Toulouse."

She proffered a delicate hand and a charming smile, *"Enchanté."* The bleak foyer was suddenly transformed, suffused with intoxicating perfume and a glowing magic.

The Marquise sat next to me in the darkened limousine as we drove to the outskirts of the city. The other three Americans, a young woman from Philadelphia and two men from Boston, did all the talking. I sat speechless, trying not to stare at the elegant face of the Marquise. I felt like a stable boy escorting a queen to a grand ball. A poor medical student, I was hardly dressed appropriately for such a splendid occasion in my old brown corduroy pants and a nondescript sport jacket.

What does a struggling student from City College of New York have to say to the Marquise of Toulouse? At the time, nothing. I feared my awkwardness and shyness would make this a one-time-only invitation.

Dinner was served in a baroque dining room filled with flowers. Her husband, a man in his early fifties, was tall and slender and wore a thin black moustache. He sat at the head of the table, smiling occasionally, saying little. His English was meager. He was most comfortable with "OK," which he had learned from an American gangster movie.

One of the guests was the inspector of police. He knew English and acted as translator when the Marquise had difficulties finding the English word. Hearing that I was a medical student, the Marquise's eyes became as bright as the magnificent chandeliers above our table.

"In America," she said, her English heavily accented and wonderfully mellifluous, "you have good medicine, *n'est pas?*" She smiled, looking directly into my eyes. I was enchanted, completely at her mercy.

"*Mon mari,* my husband, he is always tired, always tired, and," she giggled in a delightful, suggestive manner, "he wants to sleep too much."

"Does he work too hard?" I asked weakly.

"Maybe yes," she answered, "maybe no. He has to care for the vineyards." As she struggled to speak in English, she occasionally turned her elegant head to the police inspector, who supplied her with the needed English words. When their eyes met she gave him a slight smile.

The inspector was in his thirties, and he looked like an Italian race-car driver. The Marquise was a striking woman, her face reflecting nobility, intelligence, compassion, sensuality. She wore a low-cut black evening dress with long strands of pearls. Her auburn hair was up in a sweep, accented by two diamond pins. She moved her hands and arms as gracefully as a ballet dancer when she spoke, and would bring them demurely to rest on her lap when finished.

"She wants to know," the inspector said in English with a Toulousian accent, "if you can give her husband a tonic?"

"And one for me, too," she interrupted. "I am also very tired," she added coyly, "always tired."

"You don't look tired at all," I said admiringly.

"You are a gentleman to say that." For a wonderful moment there was no one else in the dining room but the Marquise and me. I swam in her perfume, but noticed that her eyes often had a melancholy look, as if she were guarding dark secrets.

The first course consisted of small gray seashells lounging on a round silver platter, accompanied by a tiny fork engraved with the Marquis's crest.

"These are escargots," the inspector told us, as he saw my puzzled expression.

I had never tasted snails, and I certainly had no idea how to eat the ugly, slimy creatures. The Marquise saw me fumbling with the small fork and tactfully said, "You don't eat snails in America?"

"This is my first time."

"Well, if you permit me, I would like to show you how snails are eaten in Toulouse, and when I come to America, you can teach me how to eat lobsters." She laughed and placed the small fork in the shell ever so delicately, expertly removed the snail, took the empty shell, emptied if of sauce, and placed it on a silver side plate. I was reluctant to eat; my mind began to list all the diseases possibly carried by snails. (Medical students have a penchant for listing things that can cause the most horrible illnesses.) But I plunged in, and much to my delight, they tasted delicious soaked in their garlic wine sauce. Then came sautéed frog legs, another new experience for me. Many other dishes followed, each served with a wine from the Marquis's own vineyards.

I noticed that the Marquis used only one hand to eat his meal, which is not the custom of Europeans, who hold the knife in the right and the fork in the left. The Marquise caught me looking at her husband's motionless hand, leaned gently toward me, and said, softly and reverently, *"C'est paralysé."*

"It is paralyzed," the inspector translated. "The doctors can't find the cause. They say it is permanent nerve damage from a mysterious cause." I was ready to list all the causes of a paralyzed hand—the Marquise had only to ask. She looked as if she were about to.

People who are not physicians have the mistaken idea that medical students are as knowledgeable as graduate doctors, and in Europe especially, the medical student is highly regarded. At that time, in 1954, to most Europeans, medical students belonged to an elite class and were treated with almost embarrassing respect.

After dinner we were served fine brandy in the study, where a fire was glowing. The Marquesa sat in a comfortable flowered armchair, her long legs crossed, her delicate chin resting on one delicate finger. The other students kept the conversation flowing as we sat in small leather chairs surrounding her. When she spoke she concentrated only on the person whom she was addressing, always perfectly poised, as if she were posing for a magazine ad.

"Toulouse is an old city, not like in your America. We have few conveniences. I want to come to America." And then she looked at me, her eyes never for an instant distracted.

"I want to come to America, to New York," she said only to me.

"I would be honored to show you New York," I responded gallantly and enthusiastically. For a moment I fantasized walking hand in hand with the Marquise on Fifth Avenue. We were alone, her husband back in Toulouse . . . the brandy, the perfume, the smell of the burning wood, the orange fire—I was intoxicated.

"Would you all like to have a tour of the chateau?" she asked.

We walked through the many rooms, and then finally went upstairs, where husband and wife had spacious separate bedrooms. It was as if she saved this little bit of intimate information for last.

Standing outside her bedroom, she said, looking directly at me, "If you want to sleep in the chateau tonight, there is plenty of room. We have no children. My husband can't." She lowered her soft gray eyes for an instant.

The Marquise saw the look in my eyes and knew I would have been thrilled to sleep in one of those Louis XV four-poster beds and be covered with a large feather down, but the other students had already declined the Marquise's gracious offer. She, too, appeared disappointed.

We proceeded down to the wine cellar which was as large as the upstairs six-bedroom area. "Would you like to see our vineyards?" the Marquise asked, "and see how we make our wines?"

"You must come next week." She offered her hand to me; it felt like silk.

The inspector drove us back to our hotel and told us, "They

want to go to America to find some good doctors because the Marquis is very ill. In America you have the best medicine," he continued.

When we arrived back at our dingy hotel I wasn't prepared to end this strange sensuous evening, and I took a stroll through the narrow malodorous streets of Toulouse, where I imagined I heard the echoes of elegant carriages carrying dark, mysterious ladies to assignations, and Toulouse-Lautrec struggling through the night in his tuxedo. On both sides of the cobbled streets ran open sewers, and I remembered something by Jean-Paul Sartre, "I love everything that flows, even the open sewers."

I began another list, this time to review the diseases that I could contact from this filthy flow, including typhoid and typhus, both prevalent in France. The sewers of Toulouse ran in narrow troughs, emptied into the Garonne river which was filled with dead cats and rats, and the drinking water in most homes was not potable. In fact, few ever dared drink water in France; only wine was considered safe. Even children drank wine and bottled water. Milk was also considered dangerous because it carried the dreaded tuberculosis, another disease that raged through France. We were forewarned not to drink the tap water or eat tomatoes bought from the colorful outdoor markets because they might be carrying this germ. The merchants "cleaned" the tomatoes by spitting on them to make them look shiny before they displayed them on the wooden slanted stands. Some of the vendors had active TB and were spitting live bacilla on the vegetables.

The following Saturday finally arrived, and I was back at the chateau, strolling with the police inspector through the vineyards. It was the end of October. The grapes had been harvested for the new wine, and the naked vines were covered with cheesecloth to protect them from the long winter frost. In back of the chateau was the winery, actually a large cave in which the grapes were mechanically crushed and the precious juices drained into giant vats. It was chilly inside the cave, and there was the smell of wine and garlic. Along one side were hundreds of empty wine bottles covered with layers of dust.

"During the war, when the *cochons,* German pigs, occupied us, we could not get the proper equipment for the vats, so we improvised," the inspector explained. "The Marquis has kept everything the way it has been for the past ten years."

"Is the wine sold?" I asked.

"Oh, no," the inspector explained. "It is used only for the house. The vineyards are too small for commercial use. Much of the remaining French nobility have their own small vineyards reserved for the family." I listened, but I was more interested in seeing the Marquise again than in touring the vineyards.

When we returned to the house a welcoming fire was blazing in the living room, exuding a sweet smell. "Those are vines they are burning," the inspector explained.

The Marquise was standing by the large Gothic fireplace with a troubled expression on her face. She still wore black, but now it seemed solemn, as if she were in mourning. "My husband is not feeling well. He will not join us for dinner," the Marquise said. "Please, perhaps you can go up and see him. Please."

I wanted to remind the Marquise that I wasn't a doctor yet but I couldn't refuse her.

The Marquis was in a large bed, a nervous Doberman Pincher lying very close by, not quite sure what to make of me. A fire was roaring in the room and the Marquis was reading *Figaro,* the French newspaper. The dog snapped to its feet. I dared not move.

"Entré, entré, cher ami. Enter dear friend. *Je suis malade.*

I am sick," he said. "It is my digestion. It's the *vents du midi*, the winds from the north. *J'ai mal au foie*. I am sick to my liver," he said. *"Le mistral* is here."

It is still the belief of the enlightened citizens of France that each year the winds blowing from the mountains bring with them "bad breezes," which cause migraine headaches, joint pains, constipation, bad temper, and in women, terribly painful menstrual periods. There were colorful signs displayed in the drug stores in Toulouse advertising special pills for special ailments brought by *le Mistral*. The Marquis complained of most of these symptoms as he lay in his bed on three large down pillows. He wore a blue silk scarf and a red silk cap. Later I was to learn that it was the same cap that his father had worn on his death bed. The Marquis apparently was dying of a mysterious, undiagnosed illness.

I examined him as completely as I could with one eye on the dog and found no abnormalities except for the hand which dangled from its wrist like a dead chicken wing.

"You better get a real doctor to see him," I told the Marquise. "I didn't find anything, but he *looks* sick enough to go into the hospital. Why not call in Professor Riviere, the chief of medicine at the college?"

"I know Riviere very well," the Marquise said. "He is a close friend of the family, but it is so late now I dare not disturb him. It may be the wind. He gets this way every year."

"The mistral does strange things to us Toulousians. More crimes are committed during the mistral than any other time," the inspector said.

Professor Riviere, chief of medicine, was the image of doctors romanticized in novels. He was tall, handsome, charming, and brilliant. He had trained at the Mayo clinic and spoke perfect English, almost without an accent. I attended his lectures every morning, sitting on the cold marble steps that served as seats for the students. It was so cold in this lecture hall that we had to wear our coats. When Professor Riviere lectured it was like watching a Shakespearean actor perform *Hamlet* or *King Lear.* I can still remember, over thirty years later, most of the material he dramatized so effectively. The few women students stared at him enraptured, in part because he swayed like a snake, and his smile was devastatingly provocative, charming, and seductive.

It was nine in the evening, and we still had not been seated for dinner. The Marquise and I were sitting at a small inlaid table playing checkers. "I have only one weakness—at least only one I can show you—and that is checkers," she said. She looked tired; small strands of her auburn hair fell over her white forehead.

"My husband is very ill," she said. "No one knows what he has. We have had him in the Cantonnal Hospital in Toulouse dozens of times and they find nothing. Riviere has thrown his hands up in frustration. I am very sad because I have no one except the inspector. I have been very lonely, very lonely." The last "very lonely" sent my heart racing.

After the tenth checker game, by 11:00 P.M., we finally started dinner, and I began to have the feeling I was in the center of an intrigue. Finally, at 1:00 A.M., I was grateful to go to sleep in one of the luxurious royal bedrooms. I heard the Marquise's bedroom door close, and I sighed with blissful relief.

At the first light I was up and dressed. I decided to walk to the vineyards. It was Sunday. The household help were invisible. I browsed through the large cave that smelled of garlic. Standing in one corner, almost hidden behind a rack of wine bottles was a small sack which contained a powder. A small handwritten label identified the substance as arsenic.

It was the arsenic that caused the air to be suffused with the smell of garlic. It was the first time I had made the connection. Once outside again, with the sack in my hands, I spotted one of the caretakers walking three Doberman Pinchers on a leash, and he approached me.

"Good morning, Monsieur. You can have some coffee in the kitchen. The chef is already up."

As I stood outside the winery my imagination took wing. Could the Marquis be suffering from chronic arsenic poisoning—the police inspector and the Marquise cleverly plotting his death so they could have each other? Was I somehow the middleman in a fiendish murder plot?

I thought of the movie, *Notorious,* with Claude Rains and Ingrid Bergman, in which she is slowly poisoned with arsenic served in milk. Could it be?

The chef was a typical Toulousian who spoke in a melodious accent, rolling his "r"s like the Italians, just as the inspector rolled his. The chef said he spoke English because, "I learned it during the war. I was a prisoner of the Germans, in prison with American airmen who were shot down over France."

He served me coffee with hot milk in a large Meissen cup with warm freshly baked croissants. "Would you like a glass of Algerian wine?" he asked.

"Not for breakfast," I told him.

"In France we have wine for breakfast, lunch, and dinner. Everyone drinks wine except the Marquise. The Marquis has to have a carafe of his own wine with each meal, and at bedtime."

As the chef continued chatting about the virtues of wine, the faint delicate smell of a familiar perfume heralded the arrival of the Marquise, who appeared wearing a long black nightgown, exceptionally beautiful and seductive—but her face was in anguish.

"My husband, he is not waking up," she said. "Come quickly, please. I think he is dead."

The inspector appeared from nowhere, and the chef and I joined him in racing upstairs to the bedroom of the Marquis. The Marquise, apprehensive and pale, remained at the bottom of the long staircase, staring upwards. The Marquis was alive but hanging over the bed, his bed clothes on the floor, and the room smelled strongly of garlic and wine. The Doberman Pincher was conspicuously absent.

With the Marquise and the inspector, I accompanied the ambulance to the Cantonnal Hospital in Toulouse. The unconscious Marquis was placed into a private room. Professor Riviere was summoned.

One of the honorary positions bestowed on French medical school students is to be appointed an *internat*. A highly competitive and extraordinarily difficult exam has to be taken by the student to advance to this rank. He is usually the most brilliant student in the class, one so gifted that even the professors hold him in great esteem. The *internat's* name was Jean Paul, from Lyon. He looked like an American from the West, with blue eyes and blond hair and a terrific athletic build. He spoke English fluently, as did many of the French students. I dared not tell him of my suspicion that the Marquis was being poisoned with arsenic by those closest to him.

I waited outside of the Marquis's room for Professor Riviere to begin his examination, hoping that he would suspect foul play. Professor Riviere greeted me with great politeness, "Ah, our American friend is still with us? Why are you here in Toulouse? You in America have the best technology in the world. We are still back in the age of Pasteur."

"You may not have the technology," I told the professor, "but you are the greatest diagnostician in the world. Have you discovered the illness of the Marquis?"

"Alas, no. It is a strange disease. We have looked for every cause; perhaps it is the wine. I suspect the wine," the professor continued. "The French drink too much wine."

"Or perhaps it is something in the wine," I slyly said.

"The Marquis makes his own wine and that is the best way. Many of the wines that we send to America are mixtures, some bad with some good. You don't often get the pure wine of the region unless of course it's a well-known vineyard like Chateau Lafite. The Marquis drinks only his own best wine."

"I had the privilege of being a guest at the Marquis's home," I told the professor, "and I was able to see where and how wine is made. Is arsenic ever used for making wines?" I innocently inquired.

"Not unless you want to kill your guests," he laughed.

"I am just wondering, because I saw and smelled arsenic at the winery of the chateau and in the Marquis's room."

"Well, we French use arsenic as a herbicide and insecticide, and it is common around the household."

I was hoping that I might have provided some possible insight into the Marquis's illness, but the professor, in his usual elegant way, bowed slightly and entered the room to perform his examination, while I waited outside, like an expectant father.

This hospital dated back to the fifteenth century and it consisted of long winding marble stairs and marble floors and medieval walls of crushed stone. A dim light illuminated the dreary-looking halls where nurses, wearing dark blue capes and white caps, fluttered about like silent birds. One of these nurses arrived with a steel cart loaded with medical instruments. During all this time I saw no trace of the Marquise or the inspector. The door suddenly opened, and Jean Paul invited me to enter into the room.

"Our American friend has been reading too many detective stories," Professor Riviere said, "but I gather he suspects arsenic poisoning, and that is a good notion. We in France often have strange happenings because we are too preoccupied with wine and *chercher les femmes.* Love is our credo in France, and we worship lovers and love affairs, as you Americans worship baseball, football, Coca Cola, and cowboy movies."

He continued to insult the American way of life as I quietly listened and watched the *grand docteur* take a pair of scissors and cut strands of hair from the Marquis's unconscious head.

"Do you know what I am doing?" he asked in a fatherly tone.

"I am afraid I am at a loss."

"Well, we diagnose arsenic poisoning by taking a sample of hair that we submit for analysis. If your interesting theory is correct, we will find arsenic in the hair, and the mystery of the Marquis of Toulouse will be solved; then we will need our friend the inspector to do some police work."

I was speechless for a moment and then said, "I only asked about the use of arsenic."

He gave me a dubious smile. "Go and have a glass of wine and come back in three or four hours. By then we will know if arsenic is found."

Making a great diagnosis was one thing, but diagnosing a possible act of attempted murder was more than I had bargained for. I was tempted to leave France immediately and return to Switzerland. Instead, I took the bus from the Place Esquirol, where the hospital was located, to the Place du Capital, which was a five-minute walk from my hotel. The Place du Capital was a large square lined with cafés. I picked one that had the most students sitting drinking coffee and wine. I decided to see this through, regardless of the consequences.

The medical lifeline of the French student was a book called the *Vademecum,* which is equivalent to the *Merck Manual.* I borrowed the precious book from one of the students in the café. The chapter on arsenic poisoning described some of the symptoms of the Marquis's illness; but on the previous page was a description of lead poisoning and *all* of the symptoms that the count was suffering from were listed. A senior medical student knows all the symptoms of diseases, even bizarre ones, because they may appear on a final medical examination. Many times students themselves think they are suffering from some of these rare illnesses. There was no doubt in my mind now that the diagnosis was not arsenic poisoning but lead poisoning, which is common in the United States, often found in children who ate lead paint which had chipped off the walls of old buildings.

I finished my cup of coffee—it tasted like concentrated mud and caffeine—and rushed back to the hospital. It was dark when I arrived at the sinister-looking corridors where I expected Count Dracula to come soaring down at me. Instead, Professor Riviere and his entourage of nurses and the *internat*, Jean Paul, rushed towards me.

"Tiens, tiens, our American diagnostician and detective. You were right, the hair contains traces of arsenic. The urine does also, but it still doesn't explain the Marquis's illness.

"Come and join us for dinner and we can talk about your wonderful country of America." I was relieved and embarrassed because I felt I had betrayed the Marquise and her fine hospitality. I felt like the *enfant terrible* who had cried wolf.

We arrived at a narrow street where cars could not pass. Our entourage walked through the cool night, and I could picture Victor Hugo or Rimbaud walking here. Again the gutter was flowing with putrid sewer matter, and in front of a small old weather-worn house were rows of women of all sizes and shapes, silently soliciting.

"This is part of our scenery," the professor said. "Our *putaine* are the cleanest in the world because by law they have to be checked each day by our clinics; otherwise, the policemen drive them away. Every neighborhood has its own; even the

Jewish neighborhoods have only Jewish whores, but don't look for them on Friday night and Saturday. They do not work then because of the Sabbath."

We arrived at a narrow dark alley off a crooked street that smelled of stale urine. It was the entrance into a medieval passageway that led to a circular staircase that snaked up into a belfry tower where a small restaurant called The White Horse was located. Once inside, the doors of the restaurant opened into a charming world of red-colored tablecloths and flowers. The red-faced proprietor met us, wearing a white apron. How well he complemented the décor.

After the fourth glass of burgundy, after we tired of discussing American politics and Marilyn Monroe, I struck up enough courage to ask Professor Riviere a question deeply troubling me: "If the Marquis is not suffering from arsenic poisioning, what about lead poisoning?"

Jean Paul, the *internat,* said to me in English, "Now that makes sense, but where does one get lead poisoning drinking wine?"

"The same way the Romans did," I said. "It is still believed by some that the fall of the Roman Empire resulted, in part, from lead poisoning. The population dropped drastically because of widespread sterility. The Romans had the first plumbing system in the world, as well as the first aqueduct made of lead. They distilled their wine in lead vats. After many years the lead crept into their wines. They suffered from chronic plumbism—lead poisoning."

"*Il est fou.* He is crazy this American. First he suggests the diagnosis of arsenic, now it is lead."

Almost everyone began to laugh; I was too crushed to join the fun. Professor Riviere was not laughing either. "The American has an interesting theory again. We don't often see plumbism in France because our children don't seem to eat the paint off the walls as in America. I think you call it "pica," *n'est ce pas?*"

At the slightest provocation, Professor Riviere hurled deprecating remarks against the United States, even as, in the same breath, he applauded our superb techniques in medicine.

I added, "Perhaps you have not diagnosed lead poisoning as readily as we have."

"That is also possible," he said.

Jean Paul said, "Maybe the Marquis is suffering from Rocky Mountain spotted fever. Perhaps one of the mosquitoes from Colorado imigrated to Toulouse and found the Marquis."

Again laughter, which convinced me to remain silent and keep my wild diagnoses to myself.

The following morning, at 8:00 A.M. sharp I was on the general medical ward with the other French medical students, interns, and residents. The medical ward smelled like a bar. The male ward was twice the size of a bowling alley, a dozen beds on each side of the large room. Every bed had its own small night table with a carafe of red wine and a thermometer. Most of the patients on this ward were suffering from liver cirrhosis after decades of wine drinking. In the center of the ward were large steel carts with medications and instruments and there was a nurses' station at the end of the room. The nurses, many of whom were nuns, wore large triangular hats that reminded me of those worn by Spanish soldiers on patrol.

The head nurse, a nun, rang a small bell and all the patients struggled out of their beds and sat themselves in small wooden chairs. They all had huge swollen bellies—they looked pregnant—resulting from liver failure. The orderlies placed a pail in front of each of the patients, as if they were cows waiting to be milked. The head nurse stood in the center of the ward and clapped her hands and announced, "The professor is arriving. Silence please. Everyone stand."

Professor Riviere appeared with his entourage of doctors wearing long white coats. He swayed to the center of the room and said, "Good morning, *tout le monde,* everyone. Today we do the drainage."

He stopped in front of each bed; without looking at the steel chart hanging from the bed railing, he knew the name of each patient and their course of treatment.

He spotted me at the far end of the ward and yelled across in English, "Come and join our walk and we will show you how we drain bellies swollen from too much wine."

All eyes were upon me as I stood by the professor. The intern took a brown tube and placed on the end of it a huge needle, a trocar. It looked like a spike. He painted the exposed swollen belly of the first patient with a red antiseptic, and it began to look like a red beach ball. The patient sat silently, not uttering a sound as the intern punched the spike into the swollen belly and water spurted out like a fountain. He then attached the brown tubing to the trocar and the other end into the pail, which began to fill. The orderlies stood by, watching the pails filling up. Soon all the patients had tubes sticking in their belly and Professor Riviere said to me in English, "It is like the fountains of Rome. It may seem primitive to you, but it works. We ordered a lead level on the Marquis," he whispered to me. "In a few days we will know if your idea is right. Would you like to try a drainage?" he asked me.

By the end of the day I became an expert on punching spikes into bloated bellies, and when I returned to my hotel my clothing was drenched with the ascitic fluid I had helped remove. Our hotel had one bathtub in the hall, which had to be reserved days in advance. I threw my pile of wet clothing in the corner of the room and desperately longed for the simple pleasure of a shower. The French had a reputation for being malodorous because there were no showers or bathtubs in most homes. Public baths were the norm of the day, and once a week many people bathed for the equivalent of 25 cents. The French perfume industry developed so illustriously for a very good reason.

I was contemplating such things and starting to think of the Marquise when there was a loud knock on my door. With a terrycloth bathrobe wrapped around me I opened it. There stood the inspector and the Marquise. They stared at me.

"We apologize for this intrusion," she said in a quiet voice. "We must speak to you. The idea of arsenic poisoning is a good one," she continued. "I have been afraid to drink the wine from the cellar for two years because I thought there was something in it. You would not know that because you are not *accoutumé*, accustomed to drinking wine. My husband, however, would become angry if I did not serve him his wine. I told him he must sell the vineyards because there was something wrong, but they had been in his family for more than a hundred years, and he insisted that there was nothing wrong with the wine. 'It is just a little flat,' he'd say. 'I'd rather die than sell the estate.'

"Please come to our house. You can bathe there and have some dinner, then we will drive you back to the hotel if you do not wish to stay the night."

She wore a simple raincoat and a scarf around her head. She looked like Martine Carole, a beautiful French actress I had been in love with for years. Did she always have to have the inspector at her side? Without her elegant clothing, the Marquise looked like a young woman in her late twenties or early thirties.

When we arrived at the chateau, the Marquise took me by the hand, leaving the inspector in the library, and escorted me to a luxurious bathroom that had Raoul Dufy painting hanging on the walls and Oriental rugs carpeting the floor. In the center stood a tall bathtub filled with scented water. On each side of the bathroom stood tall radiators covered with large warmed bath towels.

"Take your bath and then we will have a little supper, and you may stay here for the night," she whispered.

I undressed and stepped into the hot bath filled with the "perfumes of Arabia." I was in ecstasy. I would have fallen asleep were it not for one of the servants who handed me the warmed towels, a glass of mineral water, and a silk robe. I dressed swiftly in my corduroy pants, shirt, and sweater. The Marquise was waiting for me in the dining room, in silk Oriental pants topped with a red blouse. She was wearing the same perfume as the first time we met. This was the first time she was not wearing black. Some psychologists once told me that the color of women's clothing reflect their moods, and that bright colors indicated optimism. I grew optimistic, too, to say the least.

She saw me staring at her and quickly said, "Have some wine. It is not from our cellar, so don't worry."

During the dinner the Marquise's English seemed to improve with each course. "The inspector and I have for a long time suspected that my husband might be geting ill from the wine, perhaps one of his enemies—and he has many—was poisoning it, but we could not ever prove it. My husband is a de Gaullist, a nationalist who wants to keep Algeria French and not make her independent. As you may know, we French are in the middle of a war. Our Foreign Legion and the French army are fighting each day against the rebels in Algiers. My husband is a commander in the French army, but since the past few years, three to be exact, he has not been well and he has not gone to Algiers. Some of our servants have been Algerian."

"If this is so," I said, looking at the inspector, "why do you allow the Marquis to drink the wine?"

"Because, my dear American friend, we had the wine tested

dozens of times for different poisons and found nothing. We did not test for arsenic until now, and as you well know, traces are found even in normal persons. Even in America you can find arsenic traces in farm workers, but are they ever tested for lead? The Marquise and I are very grateful for your suggestion, but I want to know how lead could get into vats?"

"Well, I don't know. You are the police inspector. It's just something I read—some wild notion for which I apologize for starting. I am not a doctor yet, nor am I a detective."

"Professor Riviere said to us it was not so crazy," the inspector said.

"Well, inspector, don't you drink the wine? You are a frequent guest at this house." He must have sensed my envious tone.

"I have had early cirrhosis of the liver. I have not been allowed to drink wine for the past three years."

"Well, what about the servants?"

"They can only drink table wine. In Toulouse, it is ironic, but this means Algerian wine. The Marquis is the only one who drinks the wine from his own vineyards."

That is convenient, I thought to myself. The entire conversation seemed ridiculous and contrived. I felt I was being used, exploited, for some lovers' nest intrigue, an evil plot to kill the Marquis. The Marquise gently brushed her hand against my arm. "We really appreciate your kind concern."

She had detected the annoyance in my eyes. I wanted to leave as quickly as possible and take the next train back to Switzerland, but my adventurous soul would not hear of it. Or was it my interest in the Marquise? I felt as if I were being drawn into an irresistible maze.

I was relieved that dinner was over because I was now utterly drained. "Why don't you go upstairs? We all need some sleep," she said softly.

My head was spinning from the wine and a day of draining swollen bellies, and then there was the Marquise of Toulouse! Could I resist such a marvelous invitation?

I must have fallen asleep seconds after I pulled the covers over my head. I was always a light sleeper, and sometime in the middle of the night I heard the door slowly open and smelled that unmistakeable and irresistable perfume through the darkness. I faintly saw the outline of the Marquise, standing at the door; and then she moved silently, softly, like a cat. I heard the gentle rustling of her nightgown as she approached the bed. My heart began to pound in delicious anticipation. I feigned sleep and waited—hardly daring to breathe—for the Marquise to slip in next to me. Why care about the inspector who may be next door? When she is in my arms, I thought, I will simply accept it as a way of life in France; better yet, I will be performing a humanitarian act for this poor frustrated woman. All these thoughts raced through my head while I waited. And waited. Then she pulled my toe—a most unromantic gesture.

"I am sorry to awake you in the middle of the night," she said in that warm voice of hers, "but Professor Riviere just called. They found lead in the wine."

I felt simultaneously crestfallen and elated. She must have seen the disappointment on my face, and for a very brief moment I felt that she wanted to console me somehow, but then the inspector suddenly appeared in the room. The man followed her like a German Sheperd.

"We are so grateful to you," she said. "You saved the life of my husband. You will be our friend forever."

I told the Marquise I had happened to accidentally read the chapter on lead poisoning and that it was all nothing more than the wild guess of an ignorant medical student. She didn't believe me. Her look was one of gratitude, admiration, respect.

"Tomorrow," the inspector said, "the Minister of Health

will come to inspect the vineyards to discover how lead was slipped into the wine. It must be a diabolical plot by the Algerians to kill the Marquis. It is truly fortunate that the Marquise doesn't drink. It must be the Algerians. How else?"

I told the inspector that the bootleggers and the hillbillies who made moonshine in the Blue Mountains of Virginia commonly suffered from chronic lead poisoning because they used automobile radiators to distill corn whiskey.

The inspector listened with great attentiveness. His eyes were closed in thought. Then they opened wide.

"I know how it happened," he suddenly announced. "Of course. During the war, when we were occupied by the Germans, we could not get any materials to repair our leaking pipes and vats at the vineyards. We scoured junk yards to find what we could use. The only material available came from old cars, and like your moonshiners, we improvised. No one thought of lead. No one was aware that these pipes could ever contaminate our wine. I am sure that is the answer. That's how the lead bled into the vats!"

The following day an army of French health officers arrived and took samples of the wine. They found lead in the vats and in the bottled wine. The vineyard was closed by the health authorities until all the wine-making equipment could be changed. The poisoning was at an end.

Just as the lead had to be removed from the very bowels of the vats, so was it necessary to do the same for the Marquis. He received a form of treatment called chelation therapy, a treatment that binds the lead from a body and reverses all the symptoms of the poisoning. He improved quickly, except for his paralyzed hand, but he remained severely depressed, in part because he did not have the money to modernize his vineyards. Sadly, this gentleman, the Marquis of Toulouse, was soon forced to sell his magnificent estate, like so many of the nobility after the war, because he could no longer afford to maintain it.

When I met the Marquise at the hospital with the inspector, she threw her arms around me and said, "My dear sweet American, my brother and I don't know how to thank you. Our home will always be open to you, forever."

I blushed with embarrassment because I realized I had created a sordid intrigue that did not exist. So much for scheming lovers. The inspector was, after all, merely her devoted brother. How quick we sometimes are to assume the worst.

Many years later, when I was a busy practicing physician, I returned to Toulouse with my wife and children to show them the chateau of Toulouse on the rue Metz. It had been converted into a luxury hotel, but the Hotel Henry IV still existed. The Marquise, I was informed, now lived in Costa Brava, Spain. The Marquis had never really recovered from his severe depression. On the day they were to move out of the chateau, the Marquis went to his wine vats for the last time. He filled a bottle with arsenic and wine. He died five hours later.

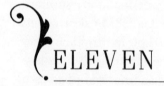

ELEVEN

The Polo Player

I MET CARL the polo player in the cafeteria of the City College of New York in the early fifties. There never was and there never again will be a college like the CCNY of earlier days. It was once the Harvard for the poor. The college cafeteria was home for students like me. We sat around the rectangular tables, weary-eyed but alive with the excitement of curiosity and companionship, until the early hours of the morning, playing chess, bridge, reading, debating the philosophy of St. Thomas Aquinas as it related to the issues of the day, especially the terrifying McCarthy era. We drank coffee in ugly, chipped mugs and smoked countless Phillip Morris cigarettes, but those were our only vices; it was before the era of marijuana and cocaine use. CCNY students were often called "Pinkies," the fashionable and painful term for those who disagreed with the McCarthy madness.

CCNY was a tuition-free college, admission gained only through a competitive entrance exam that many candidates flunked. It was actually harder to gain admission to CCNY and to survive the intellectual rigor of the place than some medical schools of many ivy-covered campuses.

Each morning to get to CCNY, I rode the subway to 137th Street. I could always tell the Columbia University students, who got off the stop before at 116th Street, by their white bucks and blue blazers, their neat appearance. CCNY students like me wore decrepit-looking clothing, and we appeared to have just rolled out of bed, eyelids drooping and faces unshaven. My wise and learned professor of organic chemistry once told us, "You guys are all cut from the same cloth."

Most of us survived by working at menial jobs while we carried a full college load. It's hard to remember that we slept at all.

Carl was an anomaly at CCNY because he wore white bucks and a blue blazer and was always clean-shaven. He was a tall, handsome man, with eyes as black as coal, a marvelous athlete as well as a brilliant student of philosophy. I was one of those struggling worn-out pre-med students whose hands and body always reeked of formaldehyde from dissecting dead cats. We and our families had escaped from the Nazis at about the same time, and we lived on West End Avenue in New York, in a neighborhood known for the "greenhorn refugees from Germany and Poland."

"I don't understand how anyone in his right mind would commit himself to ten years or more of drudgery and a disgusting life. The best years of your life will be spent studying night and day, drowning in blood, urine, vomit, and shit; then, when you are thirty years old, you may just start to earn a living. For what? To save humanity so another maniac can come around and destroy everything?"

That is what Carl kept drilling into my head as we sipped our coffee in the cafeteria of CCNY. He tried to convince me that the study of medicine was a punishment I did not deserve.

Little did he know that someday, my medical studies would save his life.

"You want to save humanity so that they can blow themselves up with an atomic bomb? You're crazier than they are! I'm going to become a millionaire and live like a gentleman while you're looking up somebody's ass."

The rest of us were poor. Carl, on the other hand, seemed always to have his charcoal gray pants stuffed with dollars. He had started a small business on his own, which was flourishing, and he owned a car—something very few of us even dared dream about. On some of the rare weekends when I was free we took trips to the "country," to Connecticut, or played tennis on the corner of 96th Street and West End Avenue, where there was a renowned tennis club, now long gone. Carl was always generous with his money, paying for everyone's beer, hot pastrami sandwiches, and the tennis court, too.

The years, as always, passed too swiftly. Carl did indeed became a multi-millionaire. Our lives took such distinct paths that we never met again until one summer day when I was invited to the polo club in Greenwich. Polo was as foreign to me as sky diving or climbing Mt. Everest.

On the far side of a magnificent lush lawn the size of a football field or two were blue tents where the polo players rested; outside the tents stood the impeccably groomed horses. In one of these tents several players sat in canvas chairs. With brilliant multi-colored silk scarves worn casually around their necks and their extravagant but groomed black mustaches, they could have been posing for a portrait of the elite cavalry guard of Nicholas II, last Czar of all Russia. Only Carl, the oldest, had no moustache. He looked the same as the intrepid and optimistic student I remembered from CCNY. His hair alone betrayed the years, it was now silvery gray, like mine. What does one say after almost thirty-five years? We embraced like brothers who had not seen one another in half a lifetime.

He didn't bother asking me what I was doing at a polo match.

"I know you became a doctor and a writer because I saw you interviewed on Tom Brokaw's news show. I was going to call you, but you know how it is. After the match we'll have dinner. We have a lot to talk about."

A few minutes later the match began, the two teams, at opposite ends of the huge green field, lined up like two dashing cavalry brigades about to attack. I shook my head in disbelief at this strange coincidence, this meeting an old friend from so very long ago. Was there a reason for this fortuitous encounter?

I watched Carl swinging his stick like a pendulum, striking the round ball smartly, man and horse as graceful as ballet dancers. I turned my head for an instant and did not see Carl fall from his horse. The crowd, in one voice, moaned concern. I ran down to the field with the emergency medical team, which had been standing by in the event of injury.

Only minutes later Carl was on his horse again, and the match continued. A stunningly beautiful woman standing next to me said, "He won't give up until he breaks his fool neck. He is too old for this." That was my introduction to Carl's wife.

They lived in one of those spacious mansions I have seen in *Architectural Digest*. They had troops of wealthy friends who shared his passion for sailing, skiing, riding, and tennis. I was introduced to these glittering worthies as "a friend from City College," a "doctor-writer pal," and as "the kid from Danzig," and he urged all his guests to quickly buy my latest book and then rush to New Haven to have their hearts examined.

In the middle of the elaborate dinner, served as if for royalty, Carl asked me if I still played tennis.

"At least three times a week," I told him.

"I have something to show to you," he said.

"Carl, can it wait till we finish dinner, please?" his wife said. He seemed not to hear her.

We walked out to the back of his mansion, where there

stood a magnificent grass tennis court surrounded by small, black, wrought-iron chairs with dazzling umbrellas. There was even a club house.

"Regard this as your private court," he said proudly.

"A long way from CCNY, isn't it, Carl?"

And then started "Whatever happened to?" for the rest of the dinner, as we carried on our own private conversation. Our friendship renewed, once a week I drove to Greenwich to play a grueling tennis match. His game was swift, accurate, intelligent; he rarely tired, even when I was on the point of collapse. We played on the hottest days, when only mad dogs and Englishmen ventured forth. After each match we sat in those delightful chairs under those delightful umbrellas, slowly sipping tall, cool drinks.

Carl usually drank several bottles of beer and the conversation often turned to medical subjects. He was looking for information—"inside dope"—some secrets that he imagined we doctors have for avoiding the terrible scourges that can afflict us as we become older. Sometimes we sat for hours, Carl always drinking and asking questions about a new drug or a new procedure. It was apparent he was much concerned about his health. He never smoked, and his diet was predominantly fish and vegetables and grains. He exercised daily, as if he were in training.

"Come on, tell me what I can do to stay alive as long as possible. I have such a great life here."

I said something to him but he did not seem to hear. He was too intense.

"I read the report in the *Wall Street Journal* that four ounces of alcohol per day is associated with fewer heart attacks and strokes," he said. He was always quoting an article about one or another recent medical finding.

"That study was poorly done," I told him. "It is a dangerous study because it will give license to a lot of people out there to drink freely. You know, Carl, patients misinterpret these sorts of statistics to their benefit. If one drink is good for your heart than surely two must be better. I think the contrary, Carl. As we get older we should drink less, much less, perhaps nothing, because the metabolism changes so much when we reach fifty. The alcohol stays in the body much longer because all of our cells have become a little sluggish, and then the alcohol can cause serious heart problems, brain damage, and for the male, impotence. One ounce of alcohol in a man over fifty is equal to four ounces in a younger person. Did you know that 25 percent of patients over 65 suffer from alcoholism? The casual cocktail hour in a place like Palm Beach means drinking for hours and suffering terrible consequences."

As I was proselytizing, Carl kept drinking, vodka and tonic now, as if I were speaking about something that had nothing to do with him. That evening the usual train of interesting and glamorous guests arrived for dinner. They were served the finest wines from his proud cellar. The dinners at Carl's home were always splendid, the food and drink and conversation complementing each other. I noticed that Carl's hand was forever holding a drink.

One week-end, when I was invited to his spacious "cottage," in East Hampton, they served breakfast with a glass of Moët, lunch with a wonderfully dry chablis, and supper with a hearty burgundy—followed of course by a rare Napoleon cognac. At the end of two days I had more booze to drink than I had had in the previous six months. It became clear to me that Carl was hardly a casual drinker. I could not understand how he could drink so much and still remain so athletic and sharp.

During one of our dinner parties at my home in Connecticut, Carl finished three bottles of wine, then proceeded to enjoy a nightcap of straight vodka. I feared for him driving home and casually mentioned that he might want some strong coffee to make the journey home safer. He looked at me with an air of astonishment.

"I never get drunk. I do like a drink or two, but I hardly let myself get to the point of being a drunken slob who is a danger on the road."

"Unfortunately, Carl, that thinking is dangerous. Your reflexes aren't quite up to par, even though you think you are sober. Why not spend the night here? Now, with our children gone, we have lots of room." To no avail.

Carl roared from our house in his new Jaguar. He was still speeding when he was stopped by a state trooper. Unfortunately, he received no ticket, despite his recklessness and the drinking. He knew the trooper.

The following week we had our usual tennis match. It was one of those torpid, hot humid July afternoons. I would have preferred dangling my legs in his pool to playing tennis. After the first set, Carl seemed to become listless. He did not dash from one end of the court to the other with his usual abandon. When we continued to play, I deliberately placed the ball in his court rather than try for the deadly drop shot. He suddenly twisted around, his racket flying wildly into the air. He collapsed. I ran to his side. He was fully conscious but his heart was racing. He refused to be hospitalized. Treated at home, ample fluids and rest helped him recuperate from his collapse, which might have been the result of heat exhaustion, except that his heart rhythm was totally irregular. I explained to him that the likely cause was too much alcohol, which can cause the heart to beat erratically. He seemed to be listening.

The summer season ended and so did my regular visits to Carl's home since there was no more tennis. In the fall he travelled to Europe to stay at the Cipriano Hotel in Venice; during winter he stayed in Palm Beach at his cottage.

When spring came, I heard nothing from him. Nor did I hear from him the next spring. When the third spring arrived I finally called his home. The phone had been disconnected. I feared the worst. Feeling concerned, and not without some guilt, I contacted one of his regular friends to inquire about Carl.

"Come to dinner and I will tell you a long story that still is without an ending." After dinner my host and his wife sat in their comfortable library where we had coffee and fresh raspberries.

"When you and Carl played tennis the last time, you remember that he collapsed. Well, he did go to see a doctor the next day. Not that he did not have the greatest esteem and confidence in you, but it was his philosophy not to mix business with friendship, especially where medicine was concerned."

For a moment I was shocked and hurt. My ego suffered. If he thought I was so competent why did he not consult me? He was, after all, my good friend. But calm reflection told me he was right. Being treated by friends has many drawbacks, and a true doctor-patient relationship is hard enough to come by without affection complicating everything.

My host continued, "His doctor told him he might have heart disease, and apparently Carl also complained of numbness and weakness of his legs. As an athlete you can understand how distraught Carl became, especially when the doctor told him that he might be suffering, on the other hand, from very early Lou Gehrig's disease, especially because he kept falling off his horse."

"Or from too much alcohol," I added.

"Strange that you should mention that, because Carl did not tell the doctor he was more than just a social drinker. You know how Carl was a controlling person and rarely listened to anyone's advice. He had to always be in charge. He started to drink more than ever. Got to the point where he could not begin the day unless he had a drink. His wife knew very well what was happening but could do little about it. She threatened to leave him if he did not go for help. Everything about his behavior began to change. The once amiable gentleman became a boor. In company he was abusive. He began to mismanage his business, made dreadfully costly business decisions. His wife consulted a lawyer, started divorce proceedings. Not only was he now constantly drunk, but he had started to abuse her physically. One morning he left the house, promising her he would seek help. He never returned again. He emptied all his bank accounts and safety deposit boxes. His wife was left without funds, except for the house, which was worth little because Carl had secretly remortgaged it at least twice. We searched everywhere for him, but never found him. His business collapsed, as expected, and his wife had to borrow money from her friends to survive. The house was sold. There was no trace of Carl. Some say he settled in a small town in Portugal; others claim to have sighted him in Rome and Paris, even in a small town in Switzerland. Still others think he may have returned to Danzig."

"Not Danzig. That I am sure of," I told him.

All in all, it was an astounding story.

"Why do you think he did it?" I asked.

"That is not too hard to figure out. It is true he was a drinker, but the threat of a divorce and having to part with perhaps half his estate was too much for him to bear. He had seen many of his friends ruined by divorce. He wasn't going to be one of them. As you know, he started from nothing. He was too proud to return there."

Several years later I received a strange call from New York. My secretary could barely understand the caller. His speech was slurred. "This is Carl. Remember me? I need some help," he said, "just a few dollars to tide me over. You know I'm good for the money."

"Where are you?" I asked.

"I am staying at the Bleecker Hotel in the Village."

"Carl, stay put, please!" I remembered the Bleecker Hotel as a decent hotel in Greenwich Village where we sometimes met while at CCNY. It was then a hangout for aspiring literary types, students, and artists. Nothing suggested it would become the flophouse it is today.

A group of dirty and wretched men were lounging about the entrance of the hotel, passing a paper bag that contained a bottle of wine. As I started to enter the hotel I heard my name called. The voice sounded familiar but it came from a pathetic man dressed in rags, sprawled on the pavement. As I walked towards him he began to crawl toward me like a dog.

"Hey Doc, I'm a little down and out. How about a ten to tie me and my friends over for a while?"

"Carl?" I asked in total disbelief.

"At your service, sir." I grabbed him by the arm to try to lift him to his feet. He was no sooner up then he fell to the ground, striking his head on the pavement.

"Now look what you've done!" one of his cronies screamed at me. "You know the Professor can't stand up no more." The sight of this once elegant and powerful man, now surrounded by pitiful and desperate souls, broke my heart. As I looked at him, caked with filth and surrounded by filth, I wanted to run away, to get away, to forget what I was looking at. I felt so helpless to do anything for him. He was too far gone, like a person in intensive care suffering from a terminal illness. I wanted to disconnect the respirator, but there wasn't one to unhook. I couldn't run away.

He awoke in a few minutes. I pulled his filthy body up

against the side of the building, and he looked at me, drunkenly, vacantly, stupidly.

"Thank you, mate. I must have hit my head against the boom."

I was with him in the ambulance taking him to a hospital where injured drunks are often brought. The resident doctor recognized Carl and was surprised that he was being brought in by a doctor.

"It's Carl again. We see him at least once a week because he either was in a fight or banged his head. Each time he is stinking drunk."

"Can't you admit him for 24 hours or so?" I asked in a pleading voice.

"Come on Doctor, could you admit him to Yale if he arrived in your ER drunk once a week? We'll clean him up and let him sleep. We have seriously ill people waiting in the ER for days to be admitted. You know that, Doctor." He spoke to me as if I were a schoolboy.

"At our hospital we have similar problems," I told him.

The resident was genuinely concerned about poor Carl's plight, but there was nothing he could do, nor could anyone.

"Are you sure that Carl's problem is all alcohol?" I asked the resident. "Is it not possible that he could be carrying another illness, like a brain tumor? When he was in Greenwich I saw him fall off a horse during a polo match, and the last few times I played tennis with Carl he had difficulty remembering the score. But he wasn't drunk when we played tennis."

The resident looked at me peculiarly: "This guy played polo and tennis and lived in Greenwich? I find that hard to believe. Are you sure it's the same guy?"

"I'm sure it is him—despite his decrepit appearance. Can you at least have the neurology resident examine him one more time and order a CAT scan on him just to be sure. I don't have privileges in this hospital, my hands are tied."

"Since you are so anxious to waste tests on him," he said, "why don't you let me put him in your car so you can drive him back to Yale where you can do all the tests."

"First of all, I don't have my car with me, and I would have to take him by ambulance. Besides, he doesn't look like he's in any shape to travel."

It was midnight when I returned to the Bleecker Hotel and found some of his cronies lying on the pavement, not far from where had I left them.

"I have five dollars for each of you, if you can tell me something about Carl."

"You mean the Professor? You aren't a cop, are you?" one of them said.

"No, I am just a doctor, and I think he is the same person I once knew in Connecticut. He was a very rich and important man then."

"We all were rich and important," one of the drunks said.

"How long have you known him?"

"Give us the fiver and we'll tell all," the oldest in the group said. Their eyes widened as I took out my wallet and handed them a twenty-dollar bill. It was foolish of me to do this on a dark street at midnight, surrounded by such desperate men. Perhaps my telling them I was a doctor gave me immunity from being mugged. They must have seen the fear in my face because one of them said, "Don't worry, Doc, we aren't going to do you no harm."

"I met the Professor a while back, in jail," the oldest one said. "He got in a fight on Mott Street. He was strong, and he had plenty of money in his pocket, but the cops didn't believe it belonged to him so they took it. I stuck close to him because he had plenty more which he hid somewhere. He had trouble walking so I helped him along."

"Yeah," one of the drunks added, "Big Jim became his valet," and they all laughed at that. "He kept telling us what a big man he was. He said he just came back from Paris where he lived for six months, and he travelled all over from bar to bar. Finally, he stayed in Spain on an island, or something, but he got bored with that."

"Did he say, by any chance, that the island he stayed at was Majorca?" I asked.

"Yeah, that's it."

After we had graduated from CCNY and before I started medical school in Switzerland, Carl and I had hitchhiked from Paris to Barcelona. There we took a cattle boat to Majorca, where we expected to stay a day or two. We stayed in an American colony called El Torino, and we both had our own exciting adventures that stretched our stay to two months. To the chagrin of our families, we simply disappeared. If it wasn't for medical school obligations, I would have stayed on and on.

The El Puchet Hotel was a charming small hotel facing the Mediterranean. Other guests included a drunken Englishman. The Englishman had just won 5,000 pounds on the British sweepstakes and for two weeks all the drinks for the guests of the hotel were on him. He was drunk from morning to night. Although he entertained us with his great wit, he made a pathetic scene sprawling over the dining room table, and Carl remarked that he would never, ever, allow himself to get to such a state, and that he would kill himself before he'd disgrace himself.

We had left for the famous Harry's bar because the hotel had become like Sodom and Gomorrah. Carl couldn't bear seeing the Englishman in that state, and neither could I. That night at Harry's bar we met George Sanders, Walter Sleznak, and Herbert Marshall, actors all, which started us on another adventure.

I wondered why Carl couldn't keep his word to never become like the drunken Englishman.

The drunk continued to tell me about Carl. "He is always in trouble. Once he walked into "21" asking for his table and they threw him out. He just stood there screaming, threatening to call his friend who owned the place and get everyone fired. He wouldn't leave until some big guy grabbed him by the neck to throw him out, and the Professor punched him in the face. He landed in jail again."

"So all this time he's lived on the streets?" I asked.

"Not always. He would disappear and come back with a fresh supply of money, but then he got worse and worse and we had to take care of him."

When I returned to the emergency room, Carl was lying on a stretcher receiving I.V. glucose. He was fast asleep. When he awoke he would be sent out into the streets again. I thought of one of my medical school classmates who was a neurologist practicing in New York. It took a great deal of convincing to get him to come down to the ER to examine a drunk.

"I promise you a dinner at Côte Basque and a weekend in Connecticut. I just want to be sure this guy is all alcohol and not something else."

The resident allowed me to sleep on a stretcher while I waited for the neurologist to arrive at six in the morning.

"This better be worth it," he said, more than a little annoyed when he arrived.

"Call it a humanitarian act," I said. "You know, like when you worked at the Albert Schweitzer Hospital." He didn't think my comments appropriate.

This ER is one of the largest in the city. Carl had been placed in one of the overnight stalls, but when we arrived at his bed in the morning it was empty. The I.V. tubing was on the stretcher; there were drops of blood on the sheet. Carl had again disappeared. We were about to leave when he returned, his fly open, his trousers wet. He staggered back to his stretcher, completely unaware that we were standing next to it. The neurologist gave me a disapproving look, but his expert eye quickly surmised that perhaps Carl was suffering from more than alcoholism.

"I am going to examine you, Carl. That is your name, isn't it?" he asked.

"It sure sounds like it."

I approached the stretcher and looked into Carl's eyes.

"Do you remember me, Carl? We used to play tennis together when we were students at CCNY. Don't you remember how we organized the strike against Professor Knickerbocker for his anti-Semitism? Howard Fast came to speak in the Great Hall for our cause? We made the front pages of the *New York Times* after we burned the fascist bastard in effigy. And the night we won the double NACC basketball championship? Remember when Warner and Roman threw the game? Remember saying that, "Honor and dignity are foremost: that is all our kind have?"

"If you say so, Doc. You look familiar. Were you on my ship?" Carl had been a petty officer on a frigate during the Korean War, while I worked as a merchant seamen on the *Mankato Victory,* a cargo ship.

The neurologist concluded his examination and ordered a CAT scan, much to the objection of the resident.

"This is the third one in three months and they're always negative," the resident lamented. "No wonder medical costs are so high." The resident was an activist who rightfully wanted to cut medical costs and only order essential tests. He was not intimidated by the malpractice threats forcing doctors to order too many tests. But this time he was wrong.

"Look into his eyes with your ophthalmoscope and you will get a surprise," the older physician said.

The resident, without saying another word, examined the back of Carl's eyes with the ophthalmoscope, then looked up and said, "His eye pressure has increased. I'll be damned. I assure you it wasn't this high the last time he was in."

"I am sure that is correct," the neurologist said. "Something has changed, so let's get the CAT scan."

My neurologist friend and I went to have breakfast in the hospital cafeteria. We tried to catch up on the past ten years while waiting for the CAT scan to be performed.

"Well, I guess, old friend, you were right to call me in. This poor bastard has something. It isn't a tumor because an earlier CAT scan would have demonstrated it. His staggering gait, his memory loss, and inability to hold his urine, his entire personality change could be explained by one thing. There is a disease you cardiologists probably never heard of. It was described after you left medical school. It's called internal normal pressure hydrocephalus. These patients have repeated normal CAT scans and normal pressures, and many are never diagnosed. Some get the diagnosis of Alzheimer's disease because the CAT scan in the advanced stages shows large brain atrophy, like Alzheimer's disease."

"What is the cause of this wild disease of yours?" I asked.

"Many times there is no cause. Sometimes it can result from repeated falls, like those suffered by your polo-playing friend. If this is the correct diagnosis he will be case number 4,001. This is a relatively rare disease, but we can ask one of our neurosurgical colleagues to perform a shunting operation to relieve the pressure in his brain and that can cure him. Does he have medical insurance?" he asked me. "Because he has to be admitted into the hospital."

I shook my head.

"Regardless, I'll get him in and get him cleaned up, and then we will see what we can do for him."

Carl stank like a rotten barrel of wine. The nurses had to

scrub his body with detergent for hours because the dirt had become embedded in the skin. His hair was matted together as if someone had poured glue on his scalp.

When I saw him the following evening he was clean-shaven, but his face looked old, covered with those small red blood spots seen in chronic alcoholics. He was lying in the bed, his hands tied to the bed railing because his body was shaking like a trembling leaf. The air was suffused with that unmistakable sweet smell of paraldehyde which was given to alcoholics when they pass into dt's. He was yelling obscenities and muttering in an incomprehensible language that only he could understand. I knew it would take a few more days before the withdrawal reaction would pass and Carl would return from his terrifying world of monsters and goblins. His return to reality would allow the neurologist to get a better picture of Carl's underlying illness.

Several days later Carl's dt's were over, and he was awake, sedated on librium to prevent him from having another withdrawal reaction. He was lying in bed quietly, still slightly tremulous, still in his twilight state.

"I am glad to see you," he said softly.

"Do you recognize me?" I asked him.

"Of course I do. You're Mother Teresa." I then knew that Carl was recovering.

The CAT scan did show just what the neurologist suspected. A wonderful example of medical detective work by an experienced doctor.

Carl had a long and trying time. Although the surgery was a success he developed many complications. The worst was a fulminating pneumonia that prolonged his hospital stay into months. As he began to recover I noticed a complete change in his personality. He underwent a metamorphosis, as if his brain metabolism had altered. He lost his previous aggressive demeanor and slipped into a peaceful lassitude, as if he were on tranquilizers, although none were given to him. The prolonged hospital stay was therapeutic for him. He spent the hours reading philosophy and ethics, and on the day of his discharge we had a long talk.

"I don't have to be a millionaire again," he said. "I was given a second chance with life. It took this horror to learn my real self and values. I am going back to start where I left off forty years ago. I have my MA in philosophy; maybe I can get a job teaching. Once you survive a brush with death everything changes." He looked me straight in the eye, as if he knew something I didn't.But I was soon to know, too.

TWELVE

The Yellow Light

THE MORNING OF February 21, 1982, was gray and dreary; I was making arrangements for a trip to Boston and upstate New York, the last obligation of the TV, radio, and lecture publicity tour I had undertaken for my recently published book. All morning I felt uneasy, restless, and exhausted. I was peculiarly reluctant to leave. Perhaps it was the comfort of Sunday morning, surrounded by my chatting and cheerful family at the breakfast table. Also, it was the kind of gloomy day that invites one to stay in, reading, watching an old comfortable movie on TV, or simply dozing before a roaring fire.

I had been booked to leave from the New Haven airport at six that evening, but since my first show was set for eight the next morning, I decided to leave earlier, so that I could arrive in Boston and settle in before night. I didn't feel like going at all. I thought of cancelling. I told my wife that I was worn out.

"I am coming down with a virus," I said. "My stomach feels upset."

"You really love to go on these tours," she said reassuringly.

"You'll see, once you get on that plane and to Boston you'll be yourself again. And in the morning, in front of the cameras, you'll be on a high—you're a born ham."

She was right of course, I always found it exhilarating to be front and center. This tour would be no different.

The day was unusually warm for the end of February. A slight drizzle started as I arrived at the airport. Luckily, I got the last seat on Pilgrim Flight 458. Waiting to board, I saw a little girl in a blue coat embrace her mother and then run out to the plane. I wondered why anyone would allow such a small child to travel by herself. I embraced my wife and daughter and felt a bit sad, and terribly uneasy. I suddenly wished I had driven to Boston, but that would make no sense: there was still Syracuse and Rochester and Buffalo. Even though these tours harvest few book sales, I really enjoy the notoriety. And while they only last a few days at a time, they offer a change from my tumultuous life in medical practice.

An experienced traveller, I always request the seat behind the pilot on these small Otter planes. Snaking myself down the narrow aisle, I caught a glimpse of some of my fellow passengers. They seemed mostly young. There was a tall black man. A mother and her son were in the seat opposite mine. The little girl I had seen in the terminal, in the blue coat, sat next to a young man at the back of the plane. There were twelve passengers in all on this flight. My raincoat was on my lap, as was my briefcase, which contained a new manuscript I was working on.

We were airborne in minutes. I could overhear the son and mother talking. "I hate to fly," the mother said. They were Californians on the last leg of their trip to Boston. Their voices were unusually loud, as if they were both compensating for deafness. It was difficult to concentrate, but I spread the manuscript on my lap. From the side window I could see New Haven Harbor, covered by an eerie-looking mist. There were two pilots. One was giving the usual in-flight instructions to the passengers, which was terribly garbled because of a defective PA system.

After we were in the air for fifteen minutes, I watched the senior pilot pull the flight lever to descend. We landed in Groton to refuel, and from the window, I spied the pilots chatting as they waited. They seemed, at least for an instant, to be arguing, or at least, disagreeing. A young woman carrying a clipboard joined them, and both pilots were satisfied with whatever they read on it. They wore gray flight suits and were in their thirties. I wondered why pilots were always so tall and strong looking, and charming. They gave me confidence and trust. They made these small commuter planes seem somehow larger, more substantial.

"Well folks, we are off again. As you all saw, we've taken on fuel because this flight started in New York. We should arrive in Boston in forty-five minutes," the senior pilot informed us cheerfully. As soon as we were airborne the windshield was covered with pelting rain. The uneasiness that I felt all day had steadily increased. I stared at the large windshield in front of me. It was no use. I had no interest in my manuscript. I placed the sheets into their folder, returned the folder to my briefcase. I sat back, trying to relax.

I began to plan what I was going to say on this next interview. Lionel Trilling once said that if you speak to the heart of your listeners you will have a large attentive audience. It made sense. But, it was impossible for me to concentrate. Instead, I began to wonder if I would die in a plane crash. After all, I had been fortunate so far, having traveled hundreds of times without mishap. Perhaps it would soon be time to give flying a little rest. Why push the odds, or my luck?

Death had not really preoccupied my mind until now, although as a cardiologist, it is a constant companion. How many times have I stood by a bedside and been a witness to the last moments of a human life? Everyone dies the same, unlike births, which are always somewhat different. The last gasp of life is a universal phenomenon, regardless of the cause or what had happened previously. Death is the end of a personality. "That's all there is folks, there's no more!" the man in the circus used to shout. Being the custodian of human lives, I am programmed to save them. This is as much a part of my brain as eating, sleeping, all those other normal functions. But who would try to save mine when the time came? Who saves the doctors, those with the highest mortality and shortest life span of any profession?

I took a comb from my jacket and began to straighten my hair, arrange my tie, smooth the blazer I was wearing, as if I were grooming for a party. I felt a strange silence permeate the plane, a kind of Sunday afternoon listlessness, when after a large family dinner, everyone returns to the living room to catch twenty winks.

I found my senses becoming more acute. I was sitting on the edge of the narrow seat poised like a runner about to break from the block. Turning my head to the rear of the plane, I saw the others relaxing, their eyes closed. They had full confidence that everything would be the same when they landed in Boston as it had been when they left. Why then, was I so jumpy, so increasingly anxious?

My eyes were transfixed by the windshield. The wipers were moving—large, thin blades that looked like long spider legs gliding back and forth, back and forth, across the glass. How could the pilots see through all the fog and mist? Then I realized that they were instrument flying.

Suddenly the wipers stopped moving while in the very middle of the windshield, like a movie that abruptly freezes a frame of the action. Quickly, in seconds, ice formed on the glass, and

I saw that the pilots looked strained as they started pulling and pushing different levers. I placed my arms in front of me. Terror was about to strike, and I felt it, knew it. Did anyone else? The woman sitting in back of me who was about my age? The little girl? The black man who was going to be interviewed for a college football team? The secretive German traveler, who held on to his briefcase as if his life depended on its contents?

First came a tinge of odor, almost imperceptible, but somehow familiar to me. The odor increased. It was not disagreeable. It increased again, and now I recognized a smell I meet each day in my office, in the hospital, in the operating room— alcohol. It covered the windshield, but the long wipers remained paralyzed. Behind me, the passengers were still in their etherized state, oblivious, comfortable, safe. The alcohol was unmistakable now, the same smell as the sponges used to clean the skin before venapunctures. Suddenly I was back in time. It was twenty years earlier, in the hospital. I was attempting to draw blood from a patient. I missed, and the needle raced through the rolling vein. I felt so bad that I said "I'm sorry to hurt you. I have to get blood from you. We have to do these tests." She was an elderly woman dying of kidney failure. The perforated vein began to swell up like a blowfish out of water. Luckily the patient knew about these things and gently said, "Just press on it, and the swelling will go down."

A little puff of smoke started to curl around the cockpit, slowly increasing, until in minutes the entire cockpit was hidden behind a thick blue miasma of death. The smoke made my breathing more and more labored. I felt like I was submerged under water, occasionally struggling to the top to gasp for air. As I write this, I am again filled with the terror of the memory of the smell. Behind me, the passengers awoke. Sleepy eyes now stared in disbelief and fear. Voices grew louder. "What the hell is going on?" Seconds later little bursts of flame appeared from the instrument panel, fire being spit by a dragon. The fire spread, licking the walls, the cockpit. I threw my raincoat at the fire. It was ablaze in seconds. The smoke increased. I began to gasp for air. I sat back and waited. It was not possible to survive much longer without fresh air.

Is this what my family felt in the concentration camp in Treblinka? The Germans didn't get me, but the gods would finally have their filthy way. What a way to die. A dirty trick to play on me. It was unfair. There is no justice. I didn't even get to see my children married, or make the best-seller list. It was like Dante's Inferno now—hot, dark, suffocating.

"How long can you withstand low-oxygen concentration in the blood," the professor asked me on the final exam, "before brain damage occurs?"

Someone shouted, "Where is the fire extinguisher?" and grabbed my tennis racket. This was a pressurized plane. We can't break a window, I thought. We mustn't. But this someone did, smashing the glass until it gave. The pilots were now festooned in flames, but one of the ghastly figures stuck his head out the smashed window as the plane suddenly dove at a steep angle. The plane began to shudder and rattle. Down, down! Death was upon us. I could see mountains. But there were no mountains in Connecticut.

These were ice-covered mountains.

I'm in Switzerland again, in the very attic where I had lived while at medical school. There is no heat or hot water in my room, just a little electric stove, and it is a frigid winter. There is a small bed and desk with my open books. Next door lives Klaus, also a student. On his desk are pictures of the Führer standing next to his father.

"Were you in the war, Klaus?" I asked.

"Yes," he answered me in German. "I was in the submarine

service. I knew nothing of what went on. My father was Hitler's friend, a close friend."

Klaus and I often shared our coffee and exchanged notes. One morning he was found dead, having jumped from the bridge in the center of town.

Suddenly the mountains were covered with a blinding bright yellow light. I squinted to see. I heard soft voices. It was so peaceful, the most peaceful moment of my entire life, absolute serenity. I was floating above the plane, an objective observer calmly watching it burn.

I must have passed out—or had I died? The plane was on the ground. We had crashed. I unfastened my seat belt, moved my arms and legs. There was no pain anywhere, only the heat and the stifling smoke. I lurched out of my seat. There was moaning and screaming now, the sounds of disaster, as I tried to run to the back of the plane. The exit door was blocked. I cleared it, then kicked it till it flew open. A tall man standing behind me dove out of the open door like a swimmer diving into a pool. Lying at my feet was the little girl with the blue coat, shrieking. Her face was covered with blood. I grabbed her by her coat and dragged her out with me as I struggled to leave the burning plane. I touched ground. It was hard and icy cold. It must have snowed, I thought. I dragged her along the ice, away from the blazing plane.

"Stop pulling me," she screamed, "you are hurting my back!"

"Everything is okay, you're fine," I said, the doctor speaking.

Suddenly one of the pilots appeared, black as charcoal, weaving from side to side as if he were drunk. His leg was ripped and bleeding.

"Get away from the plane!" I heard someone shouting. Passengers were crawling, staggering away. The little girl in the blue coat was suddenly able to stand up and walk. A young woman, arms outstretched before her, was feeling her way.

"I can't see!" she screamed. I took her arm and escorted her away from the inferno. Her face was wet and red, her eyes swollen shut. We moved slowly, a grotesque march from hell. Now a terrible explosion, as if planets had collided. Then an ugly pile of acrid smelling burning debris was all that was left of Pilgrim Flight 458 headed for Boston. That same sense of utter peace I had experienced when the conflagration began, returned. Still there was no pain, even though I knew I was injured. There was only numbness. My knee was swollen to the touch, and my ankle looked black. We could all feel the warmth from the burning plane. Am I still alive? The young woman placed her arm in the mine.

"I'm so scared. Please! I don't see anything. Where are we?"

"You are fine," I reassured her. "We are saved. Don't worry. I'm a doctor. I will take care of you."

"Are you really a doctor? Oh, thank God! God sent you to me."

What I thought at first was frozen ground was a lake, a frozen lake on a warm day. Somehow we had to cross this icy body of water to safety. I strained my eyes to spot the shore. I thought I saw it a long way off. If the ice were to give, the blind girl clutching my arm with all her strength would pull me down, and I too would drown. I could have left her to wander off by herself, to save my own life. I was well enough to make it to the shore. But how could I leave her? I had never abandoned a sick person in my life, surely I couldn't then.

"We have to walk very carefully," I told her softly. "We're on a frozen lake, but the ice seems spongy, wet, walk carefully, step carefully."

Her grip on me grew still tighter. She took small steps, brought her feet down daintily, as if she were walking on eggs.

"Just pretend that we are walking in the park on a nice, fall day and that everything is safe and beautiful," I said softly. "We are lucky to have survived the plane crash. You will tell your grandchildren of that one day."

Our stroll continued, like two lovers arm in arm. Each step could mean the end of us both. I felt the patches of soft ice move slightly below our feet, but the lake, thus far, had remained frozen despite the warm air. We strolled on. This was worse than the crash because we were so close to surviving. Yet stretching far before us was the frozen lake we had yet to cross.

The plane, we were later told, had crashed right in the center of the lake. I never felt the impact of the crash. The plane slid and sailed 1,000 feet across the ice before the nose finally, and gently, dipped into the lake, a huge bird taking a drink. One of the wings of the plane had broken off. We approached it on our promenade across the lake. The bird's wing lay flat on the ice, smouldering. I watched it slowly begin to sink and disappear below the surface. It hissed. I didn't tell my blind escort what was happening, but she heard the terrifying hiss, the swishing sound as the reluctant wing was drawn to its icy grave.

"What was that?" she asked in panic.

"It's the wind, nothing more. We'll be on the shore soon. We'll be safe."

Now I could clearly see the shore. On the banks of this lake of death were some young boys, standing, watching, but no one else to help.

"Walk towards the other edge!" they yelled. "It is all melted here."

We changed our course like mariners sailing the dark sea. Now I saw that others had already reached land. They urged us on. We approached shore, and the ice became soft as pudding. It reminded me of how I once crossed the streets in New York as a child. First stepping on the ice on the edge of the sidewalk and then suddenly being in water, slush. Three young boys came to the very edge of the lake with their arms out-stretched. We were entering water now, the young woman clutced me ever more tightly as, with each step, we began to sink. The icy water reached my thigh, but it felt like hot moss. One more step. Safety was five feet away. I threw her with all my strength, and the three boys grabbed her by the arm, pulled her out. I struggled to get to land, the water almost reaching my shoulder. Another step. Another. The boys had me. A mightly pull.

Soaking wet, I began to feel terribly cold. We walked, the three boys leading us through the thick vines. Surely this must be a beautiful spot in the spring: yellow forsythia in full bloom, framing the lake. We then climbed over a barbed-wire fence, and now we were on the road. I looked back. We had cheated the Lady of the Lake.

One of the pilots was lying on the ground, a terrible pile of charcoal, unconscious.

"He is the doctor!" someone yelled.

I struggled over to the charcoal body. He was still alive. What did they expect me to do? Here? Now? It took twenty dreadful minutes for an ambulance to arrive. Isolated from the world, we had crashed in the Scituate Reservoir in Rhode Island, a body of water that had rarely been frozen before, no less on a day when the temperature was 50 degrees.

They packed me in the ambulance with the burned pilot, the blind young woman, and the mother and son from California, who both suffered bone fractures and head injuries. In their haste, one of the ambulance attendants forgot to close the back door, and as they sped off we were in worse danger than on the ice. The gods apparently were still not satisfied. We began to slip towards the gaping hole left by the open door, like children in a park on a slide. I held fast to the stretcher nestling the unconscious but groaning man. The others were screaming for the ambulance to stop, but they did not hear our desperate plea! I grabbed a bottle of saline solution from a rack and threw it at the window separating us from the driver. He turned his head towards us and was horrified to see us hanging on for our very lives. He stopped. The door was made fast.

For the rest of the trip, as the ambulance raced toward Rhode Island Hospital, I felt helpless trying to gives some comfort to this poor man who was burned over at least 75 percent of his body. This man was a great hero; so was his co-pilot. He had brought the plane down while his body was encased in flames, somehow steering the plane with his head outside the window. He will forever live in a place of special honor in the hearts of the surviving passengers of Pilgrim Flight 458. We soon realized that a miracle had occurred for those of us who had survived. The pilots, Thomas Prinster and Lyle Hogg, received awards for their heroic acts. We would remember them as supermen who ignored their own agony and terror to stay at the controls to skillfully land a blazing plane full of passengers totally dependent upon their heroism for survival. Is there anything greater than the saving of life?

We finally arrived at the emergency room of the hospital. It had been the longest ride of my life. I walked out of the ambulance against the warning shouts of the emergency-room staff.

"Don't bother with me," I said, "I'm fine." I walked towards the cafeteria while other patients looked on as if I were totally mad.

"Doctor, you must sign in and be examined. You just survived a plane crash!" the nurse shouted at me.

I gave her a derisive smile, and said, "All I want is a hamburger. I haven't had one in years, since I've been on that damned low-cholesterol diet."

I was hungry. Famished. I felt as if I hadn't eaten in weeks.

The adrenalin was overflowing. I ate three hamburgers in two minutes and then called my wife.

"Don't get worried, you probably heard of the crash. If you didn't, turn on the radio. Come and get me. Bring a coat, a hat, and a bottle of scotch"

When my wife and daughter arrived, I was lying on a stretcher being examined by an intern. They did not know what to expect, and both burst out in tears of joy when they saw that I was in one piece. Much to the dismay of the emergency-room staff, I grabbed the scotch and drank to my heart's content. My knee was injured, but I refused to stay in the hospital. As I was leaving the emergency room, Jeremy Geidt, a Shakespearean actor from the Yale Repertory Theater, approached me to thank me for pulling his daughter Sophie, the little girl in the blue coat, off the plane. The press swarmed, vultures lusting to hear from me about the crash, especially because I was a doctor. I did get my day on TV, and the coverage was better than my publishers ever dreamed. Coast to coast, on every network, in the morning, at night, I was interviewed and quoted, particularly, "It was like Dante's Inferno." Every newspaper in the country, it seemed, and in Canada, had a paragraph about the crash and the miracle of the survivors. Special religious services were held in my synagogue. All sorts of religious persons called and wrote me, asking, begging for interviews. Hundreds of letters and well wishes arrived each day. Just walking on the streets or going to a restaurant I was greeted like a celebrity. Almost everyone wanted to hear the most minute details of the plane crash. "And then what happened?" became a refrain. But some shunned me. "Don't tell me, I cannot stand hearing of it." I learned more about my fellow humans in the following days than I had in a life time. So many prayed and wished me well. Others felt me to be a pariah. And then there were still others who appeared jealous of my experience. Perhaps they wished to leave the mundane, to have a "crack at dying," a chance for publicity, fame? Little could they ever dream of the absolute horror of it all.

I took a long overdue vacation from my practice. My knee was badly injured, and I limped around in an ace bandage. I consulted a physician who prescribed pain killers which I quickly threw away, and I had one physical therapy session. What I needed most, and did not receive from the medical profession, was a kind word of understanding. Instead, one doctor said, "This is a minor injury. You will be disabled for several months, and don't be disappointed if you can't play tennis again. Swimming is much better for you anyhow. You're getting too old to play tennis. You should know all this, being a cardiologist." Tennis had been one of my grand pleasures in life, which only another athlete could really understand. The tennis racket had even saved our lives when it was used by one of the men to break the windows. He was a flight engineer, and we were fortunate to have him with us. Who else would have thought of breaking windows in flight? I was being treated coldly like a physician and not sympathetically like a patient, which I resented.

I consulted a neurologist to be certain I had no neurological damage to my brain. I had been a math major, and I tried solving some tough problems in calculus, which went well. I was embarrassed to tell the neurologist that during the height of the crash I had seen that famous bright light that many people describe seeing after having died and been resurrected. One of my colleagues checked out my cardiovascular system. It was normal. Yet I did not feel normal. I felt separated from the world, a visitor, an observer. Once my father had given me boxing lessons, and then I had been matched up against another boy. I had been beaten up miserably and had staggered out of the ring, dazed. That is how I felt for weeks, in a crepuscular state of utter peace. My wife told me how nice I was now, like when we had first met. "You let me help you," she said. "You don't fight. You are so agreeable, instead of being your usual aggressive, determined self." I heard my words come out, clearly intelligible, but they didn't sound like me. Whenever I looked up towards the sky, I whispered, "You didn't get me yet!" Whenever I saw a small plane fly by, I said, "Good luck to you up there." People made me feel that I had been chosen to survive. The nuns of my hospital, St. Raphael, kept saying that I was meant to do more good. The rabbi of my synagogue said that I had been tested. I assumed I had passed the test. Anyway, I was surely the luckiest man alive.

"How is it possible," the federal investigator asked me, "that you did not get one burn on your body when you sat immediately behind the flaming cockpit? The flames reached your seat. In fact, the woman who sat behind you was burned to death. It took days to identify her body." These were among many unanswerable questions—for example, why had the reservoir been frozen? It had not been for as long as the natives of the area could recall. All these questions did unnerve me to a degree. I am a scientist and had difficulty accepting that any masterplan for my survival existed in heaven. God had too many other agendas to be concentrating on me, I told the rabbi. But for his great and sincere concern, I contributed to the synagogue, and to the church, too—to cover all bases, just in case.

In the weeks following the plane crash my appetite began to fail, and I developed many unpleasant intestinal symptoms, which I attributed to a psychosomatic response. I consulted a psychiatrist who felt that my symptoms were part of a post-traumatic episode that would improve with time. They didn't. My knee was cured, and I was back to playing serious competitive tennis, but I tired more easily and lost more weight.

Doctors are notorious for making the wrong diagnosis on themselves and rarely see another doctor until things really became critical. My patients kept telling me that I looked terribly tired and was losing too much weight, that perhaps I should see a doctor. When my libido vanished like the wind, it underlined my problems.

"It is all part of the post-traumatic syndrome," the psychiatrist reassured me. "But, play it safe. Why not get a good physical examination?" he suggested.

Many doctors minimize their symptoms and try treating themselves, which often ends badly. Many doctors feel they don't wish to disturb their colleagues with their mundane problems and simply don't bother to get medical attention. Rarely do doctors go for a thorough physical. They dislike professional courtesy. I was one of those physicians. I consented to see a physician. My wife accompanied me for a "good examination in one of those professional centers in New York." After three hours—two hours and forty-five minutes waiting, and fifteen minutes actually being examined—I met with the doctor for my results.

"You are a physically healthy man and should seek some psychiatric help to help you get over that horrible event. I have a friend who specializes in plane-crash victims. Why not give it a shot?"

I received a bill for six hundred dollars and a beautifully written report bordered with gold leaf.

I still felt hardly any psychiatric effects from that memorable event. I slept well. I wasn't depressed. I was, however, continuing to lose weight and suffer from gastrointestinal distress and felt constantly bloated. I had no real fear of flying, but I did develop a sense of general cautiousness. For example, I always looked for the exit in the cinema and at restaurants, and I took extra care in driving my car. What could possibly happen next? A mugging? A car crash? A malpractice suit?

Hospital corridors are notorious places to get sidewalk consultations. I casually asked colleagues about these non-specific symptoms and received casual answers.

"Why not come in and let me do a work-up on you?"

I decided to do my own work-up. A stupid thing to do. "The doctor who treats himself is treating a fool," some wise man once said. First, I had a gall bladder examination performed, which was normal. Then I asked my radiology colleague to do a full GI series. I went to the X-ray department that same afternoon and read my own X ray.

It was a peculiarly unnerving sensation looking at my own insides. What I saw made me feel sick to my stomach. My entire small bowel, instead of showing nice long tubes of intestine, looked something like a Pollock painting, spots and flecks thrown on the canvas. It was the classical picture of a bowel seen in a variety of illnesses such as Hodgkin's disease, or cancer. I had been able to conquer almost everything in my life, including escaping from Gestapo headquarters, a disaster at sea, a plane crash, but this one was too much. I was petrified. Without a lost moment, I took the X rays and headed right into the office of one of my expert friends, Dr. Robert Aaronson. I wanted a diagnosis, and now!—just what any other patient would expect, I had a right to expect.

"Bob, take a look at these and tell me what's up, please."

He took thirty seconds and said, "It's lymphoma, most likely, but it could be a variety of malabsorption syndromes." Which meant that whatever I did eat was not being absorbed because the bowel was sick, very sick, which was why I was losing weight and felt bloated all the time. I was actually starving, suffering malnutrition with a serious vitamin deficiency. That was the reason I tired so quickly, and why, in the morning, my gums would bleed after I brushed my teeth. Naturally, I had thought I needed a dentist. In fact, the bleeding gums were symptomatic of scurvy because I was not absorbing vitamin C.

"We will have a biopsy done," he said, "as you know."

"An intestinal biopsy?" I asked, shaken.

"That would be the most direct."

"What is the prognosis these days with lymphoma of the bowel?" I asked.

I had been too busy being a cardiologist to keep up with this uncommon cancer of the bowel.

"Hard to say, three to five years with chemo, sometimes, not often, there is a cure. Aren't you jumping the gun?" he said. "We don't even have the diagnosis."

"At least I know I'm not cracking up," I told him, "as that ass implied in New York. No wonder people are suing the hell out of us."

The following morning, a pleasant warm summer day, I made my way into the hospital, as on any other morning, through the emergency room, and then the long walk to the X-ray department. My face is well known around the hospital. I greeted the guards, clerks, nurses, doctors, orderlies, barbers, newspaper man, electricians—all the men and women who run the hospital and help it run.

This morning was however different, like no other morning of my life. I now fully shared all the fears and loneliness of all the sick patients who walked through, or are wheeled through, those corridors. I tried to keep that same morning look of a confident doctor rushing to get to the wards to tend to his patients. I don't know if anyone noticed anything different.

I did not tell my family what I was up to this day. I wouldn't until I knew the diagnosis. If the diagnosis was lymphoma of the bowel, a dreadful life lay ahead of me. I had no contingency plan for this. I could not feel worse than I did that morning. Having faced death before, I was no better prepared for this new challenge than the first one. One of my colleagues, Dr. Phil Felig, a professor of medicine, a world-renowned diabetes expert, and a very religious man, said to me, "You are being tested again, like Job."

"How many times do I have to be tested?"

I was lying on a cold steel table in the X-ray department, reading a book by Stephan Zweig, when Dr. Aaronson arrived.

"How do you feel?" he asked.

"Like on a tennis court when I'm five games ahead," I lied.

He carried a long black case that looked like it could contain a violin. He opened it and removed a long tube of some thirty inches coiled like a rattlesnake with an ugly head.

"Is it alive?" I joked.

"It gets life once it crawls into your gut. Do you want some local anesthesia."

"Only if it's laughing gas."

"Well, then, full steam ahead!"

The long tube was gently inserted into my mouth. I decided to concentrate on a marvelous time in my life: Majorca, Spain, 1953.

"As soon as you feel the tube in back of your throat swallow as fast as you can."

How many times had I said the same thing to patients when I was a resident? I was afraid that I might vomit all over him. Instead, I daydreamed that I was again in Harry's Bar in El Torino, and I was sitting at a table with a beautiful young woman from Copenhagen. It was a glorious night. At the next table were famous and familiar faces: George Sanders, Herbert Marshall, Betty MacDonald, and a tall powerfully-built man with a gray beard, Ernest Hemingway, to whom I had been introduced by my Danish friend.

"Are you here for your health, doctor?" Hemingway said laughing. "Come and join us."

"I'm a medical student, not a doctor." I said.

"You mean you know all about illness now the way you never will again. I have high blood pressure," he said, "and diabetes, and I like doctors."

I felt the tube in my gut, and Dr. Aaronson instructed me to turn my body on my right side and swallow like I was eating spaghetti. The intestinal biopsy was about to begin.

"I'll hate spaghetti from now on!" I said, with a voice that came from another person.

"So, you read your book. It takes two hours." Dr. Aaronson said, and left.

I lay on my side and closed my eyes as I felt that wretched explorer invading my gut, and smiled as I returned to Majorca. We were invited to have coffee at a villa in Formento, on the other side of the island. A round full moon was directly overhead; someone played the guitar, singing Spanish music. I had come for a two-day visit between semesters and had stayed for two months with my friend, who was a well-known Danish poet. We swam off the white smooth rocks in the tepid Mediterranean and explored the caves that were only accessible when the tide was low.

After the first hour was done, I rose from the uncomfortable table as the doctor stood behind the fluoroscope to see the position of the snake inside of me.

"We are almost there," he said, like the navigator of a ship. "Only a few more inches. You can go back to your reverie. I bet this is the first time in years that you have been suspended like this. Time to think and plan. A man needs such time."

"I think quite well, Bob, in the comfort of my study, thank you."

I actually felt the tube inch down into my gut. What horror was this invader going to find in the darkness of my bowel? I

began to feel warm. At first I thought the air conditioning had
shut down. When I began to perspire profusely it became clear
that the tube had coiled and caused terrible cramps. The doctor came in and saw that I was pale and wet.

"Cramps, eh? Turn gently on your back over to your side.
That sometime moves it along."

"Can I have some water?" I asked. "I am dry."

"You can't, because then we will have to start again."

"Forget the water. I'll stand the cramps."

The only other time I felt so dry and thirsty was when
standing in the sun, the torrid sun of the Negev desert. I had
gone to Israel with my family. Out of sheer madness and a
sense of adventure, I had decided to drive from Israel to Cairo
across the desert, by way of the Suez Canal. Sadat had made
peace with Israel and the borders where now open. Unfortunately, not all of the Egyptians were as forgiving as the late and
great Sadat. They had refused to let us cross into Egypt and
had detained us at the canal. We had to stand in line for five
hours in the sun as the Egyptians pointed bayonets at us. My
daughters and wife had been amazingly sturdy, while I had felt
so dry and hot that I was sure I would collapse. They had
refused us water or shelter from the heat until they were convinced we were just tourists. That was how I felt lying on the
table—parched and afraid.

The tube finally found its mark, and with one quick twist
and pull the biopsy was successfully taken. When Dr. Aaronson
began to remove the tube from my throat, I felt like the man
in the circus who swallows the sword and slowly withdraws it
from his throat. It was the most marvelous sense of relief. And
that first glass of ginger ale was heaven sent.

By late afternoon I was back in my office, reading my mail,
answering telephone calls. I felt a sense of great accomplish-
ment.

Sleep was not possible that night, and I realized more than

ever before how much agony patients must undergo waiting for biopsy results. "We will call you as soon as we hear." So many times I have said it. I'd never say it again quite the same way.

Morning finally came. I was in the pathologist's office. He was examining the slide with Dr. Aaronson.

"The bowel is destroyed; the villi are gone," he said. "No wonder you couldn't absorb anything, and that is why you always felt so bloated. Here, take a look at yourself."

I had no desire to see the slide, but I looked and saw the denuded surface of the bowel specimen.

"Maybe it got burned in the plane," I said, trying to joke away my rising panic. "What the hell is the diagnosis?" I then yelled, finally breaking. "Is it lymphoma?"

"I can't be certain," the pathologist said. "It is a destructive process of some kind."

"Stain it with India ink," Dr. Aaronson said, "just to be sure."

The specimen was stained and we looked again. A broad smile came over the pathologist's face. "It is swarming with giardiasis. Millions of them have been feasting on your bowel."

At that moment, I witnessed the essence of good medical detection. Dr. Aaronson had the intuition to do one more thing, to stain the slide with India ink. Luck was on my side again. If he had failed to identify the parasites in my gut, I would have been treated for a different illness and not survived.

Giardia is a parasite commonly found in contaminated well waters and food, in places like Switzerland, Russia, and throughout the United States. I must have contracted the parasite on one of my many exotic trips, eating food from an open market—something I now would never dare do.

I was given a medication called Flagyl. In less than ten days, my appetite returned and I began to gain weight. My fatigue disappeared and I felt more alive than ever in my life. The diseased bowel, free from the parasite, began to regenerate and returned to normal: another miracle of nature; other organs of our bodies can do the same.

I consented to have the doctors present the case of the sick bowel at grand rounds at the medical school. Weeks later the pathologist's office was swamped with stool specimens and water testings, looking for the giardia.

I have become such an expert on this illness that I test patients' stools all the time if they present the bizarre symptoms so well known to me, and each year I diagnose one or two cases of giardiasis.